HOW TO
PRACTISE POPULATION
MEDICINE

Titles in this series

HOW TO PRACTISE POPULATION MEDICINE

J. A. MUIR GRAY

Consultant in Public Health

Director, Better Value Healthcare Ltd

OFFOX PRESS
Oxford, UK

First published in 2013

www.offoxpress.com
books@offoxpress.com

© J. A. Muir Gray 2013

A CIP catalogue record for this book is available from the British Library.

ISBN: 978-1-904202-08-0

Published by Offox Press Ltd for Better Value Healthcare Ltd

Index prepared by Laurence Errington, Edinburgh
Typeset by Anne Joshua, Oxford
Printed and bound in Great Britain by Berforts Information Press, Eynsham, Oxford.

The author and publishers are grateful to Erica Ison, Anant Jani and Nicolas Philippakis for valuable editorial assistance.

Contents

CONTENTS

Preface

'One damn thing after another' – that is how a caring and conscientious doctor described the new waves that had hit him since finishing training – evidence-based medicine, quality improvement, medical management, safer medicine, and personalised medicine, to name but the main tsunami. These have been very important but they have not created an immutable model of medicine. More waves are building up and one of them, about to break, is the clinician's responsibility to and for the population served.

This is one of the first books to be written about population medicine, in which advice has been given about how to introduce the concept and put it into practice. The learning objectives that can be achieved solely by reading are, however, limited. One of the classic books about clinician leadership lists 'three domains', of which only one – the cognitive – can be strengthened by reading:

- cognitive – knowledge and intellectual skills;
- psychomotor – physical skills;
- affective – feelings and attitudes (1).

The physical or psychomotor skills involved in leadership are not particularly important, although it does help if one is able to control excessive displays of emotion and it is essential that the emotional aspect of change is not overlooked. However, this book has been written to help develop leadership in 21st century medicine, surgery, rheumatology or pharmacy. The term medicine is used to describe the work of any clinician and not solely the work of physicians. Those who pay for health services, whether they be governments or insurance companies, desire high-value population healthcare. Although they can be helped towards this goal by public health professionals, they will not be able to succeed without the help of clinicians who have the knowledge, skills, and culture to care for populations as well as individual patients who are referred or self-refer.

The 21st century is the century of both personalised and population medicine.

J.A.M.G.

References

1. McKimm, J. and Swanwick, T. (2010) *Clinical Teaching made Easy.* Quay Books, London.

I

POPULATION MEDICINE – A NEW RESPONSIBILITY FOR THE 21ST CENTURY

This chapter will:

- focus on resource constraints, particularly the finite resource of clinician time;
- explain why clinicians feel their sole responsibility lies with the patient in front of them, a situation that arose from an era when the patient paid the doctor directly;
- describe how that relationship changes when healthcare is funded by the whole population, including people who have needs the same as those who are being treated but who have not accessed the service because of reasons outwith their control, such as language difficulties.

By the end of the chapter, you will have developed an understanding of:

- the changing responsibility of the clinician, particularly the doctor, in an era in which healthcare is funded by the whole population and not just by the patients who consult doctors;
- the dual responsibility for clinicians who manage services;
- the new responsibility of the clinician to and for the whole population and the actions they need to take to discharge that responsibility.

The traditional responsibility of doctors

Since Hippocrates, the traditional responsibility that doctors have felt to the patient in front of them either on the other side of the desk or lying in bed. This responsibility entailed complete loyalty to the individual patient, and a commitment of resources without consideration of cost.

However, in practice, clinicians have become accustomed to limiting the use of one resource to individual patients in order to ensure that is available to all. This finite resource that the clinician limits so that all patients might benefit is time. If a clinician did not limit the time given to one patient, there would be no time for other patients – indeed, clinicians would rarely get home. This practice has gone on for years despite the knowledge that not only many of a clinician's patients want more time but also that some patients would report a better outcome if more time had been invested in their care. It could be argued that clinicians have not rationed their time with sufficient rigour and, as a consequence, have suffered burnout, a problem that will become more common as the pressure on resources for healthcare intensifies.

Deriving greater value from resources

Although time is finite, the benefits of face-to-face time can be enhanced, for example, by using online resources to extend the consultation. Although money is also finite, unlike time it cannot be extended in the same way. Money is inelastic: money spent on one patient cannot be spent on another. Thus, if care is to be extended to patients other than those already being seen by a busy service, greater value will need to be derived from existing resources. This represents a new challenge, entailing new responsibilities for clinicians.

What are the new responsibilities of the clinician who must continue to remain focused on the needs and demands of an individual patient but must also take account of patients not yet in contact with the service?

How do these new responsibilities relate to the traditional responsibility of doctors?

The changing contractual position of doctors

In the 20th century, it was argued that the doctor's responsibilities were to the individual patient in a consultation and to that patient alone. Until 1948, doctors in the United Kingdom received their income directly from the patient sitting in front of them. This simple contractual arrangement is shown in Figure 1.1. For doctors in some other countries, this is still the contractual position today.

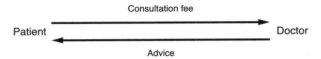

Figure 1.1 The 'direct' contractual arrangement between doctor and patient

However, with the founding of the National Health Service (NHS), the contractual relationship between doctors and patients changed (see Figure 1.2). People were no longer prevented from accessing care by its cost because the resources for care were provided by the whole population. Within the population providing the resources for care, some people:

- are patients already in contact with the service;
- have the condition (i.e. are in need) but have not yet made contact with the service;
- are healthy and will never develop the condition (i.e. not in need).

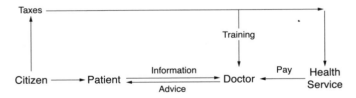

Figure 1.2 The new contractual relationship between doctors and patients

With the exception of the United States of America, this contractual arrangement exists in every developed country, although it is possible that the USA is now on the way to complete coverage of its population.

However, in the NHS, this change in contractual arrangement had disadvantages.

Some doctors no longer acted as if the 'customer was king' and treated patients with less respect.

Few doctors regarded themselves as the stewards of NHS resources and acted merely as the dispensers of resources. One medical manager remarked 'It is as if doctors were writing a cheque in the supermarket but thought that their bank was going to pay, not their own account.'

Medical management – responsibility and accountability for a service

In the last decade of the 20th century, new responsibilities for doctors were articulated – responsibilities for patient safety, quality of care, and resource management. However, many clinicians were unwilling to accept the responsibility for managing resources, leaving only a small proportion of clinicians to become medical managers. Of those clinicians who accepted the role, most were part-time; however, some became full-time medical directors or chief executives of a hospital (see Figure 1.3).

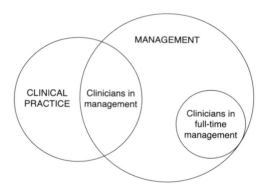

Figure 1.3 The relationship of clinicians to resource management

Population medicine – accountability to and for a population

In the 21st century, the responsibilities of a doctor continue to include loyalty and commitment to the well-being of an individual patient and to the quality and safety of the care they provide. However, these responsibilities are now complemented and supplemented by a new responsibility, a responsibility to the population that provides the resources for care.

The population providing the resources for care contains the patients who are already being treated, but for every long-term condition it also includes other people with the condition who have not yet been referred. Furthermore, the population which made the decision to allocate the resources for healthcare has done so having decided that those resources will produce more value from healthcare than if they were invested in education, state pensions, defence, or any other public service.

> *With resources always being limited, by choosing to implement one option, there is a benefit forgone as resources are then not available for other options. The lost benefit from the next best use of the resources is the opportunity cost.* (1)

The good management of resources by a medical manager is of obvious benefit to the population but population medicine entails more than resource management. Clinicians in the 21st century are expected to act as the stewards of the allocated resources, and to become conscious not only of the people who could benefit from healthcare or who are already in receipt of this benefit, but also of the 'benefit foregone' by the whole population such as the education of children or the amelioration of poverty.

The concept of stewardship has a long history: originally it concerned the administration of an estate on behalf of the lord of the manor. More recently, the concept carries connotations of a deeper responsibility that has arisen from its use in the context of environmental sustainability, for example:

> *Stewardship is to hold something in trust for another.* (2)

> *The stewardship concept demands that we constantly ask the question: will the resource be in better shape after my stewardship?* (3)

In parallel with calls for a broader perspective to be taken in clinical practice, one that takes into account not only the patient's clinical condition – personalisation – but also the patient's values and the environment in which they live – contextualisation, a broader perspective is required when considering a health service with responsibility for and accountability to not only the patients in contact with the service – the traditional role of the clinician as medical manager – but also the whole population of people in need, as well as an accountability to the population that has provided the resources for care (Figure 1.4).

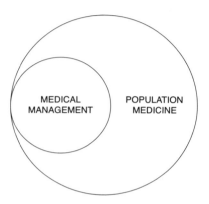

Figure 1.4 Population medicine embraces medical management

Seven actions to improve the health of populations

In the first decade of the 21st century, the focus of management and leadership development has been on managing an institution, either a health centre or a hospital. The emphasis on quality improvement, on making care more effective, and on safety (see Box 1.1), also focused around institutions, has been essential, but it is not sufficient to meet the challenges of the 21st century.

Clinicians of the 21st century have a responsibility not just to the patients who happen to have made contact with their service but also for all the people whose needs could be met, directly or indirectly, by their service. In addition to achieving high levels of quality and safety, there are seven actions that need to be taken to discharge this new set of responsibilities and improve the health of populations (see Table 1.1).

The first three of these responsibilities could be seen as an extension

---

Box 1.1 The Better Value Healthcare Bookshop

In the Better Value Healthcare Bookshop[1], there are more than 30 books on safety and about 100 books on quality improvement. For medical management, these books are essential; for population medicine, they are necessary but not sufficient because this approach necessitates many actions other than those relating to the delivery of services to higher standards of quality and safety. Key texts for each topic are listed below.

Books on safety
Patient Safety by Charles Vincent
Understanding Patient Safety by Robert Wachter

Books on the theory of medical errors and accidents
The Human Contribution by James Reason
Complications by Atul Gawande
Safety and Ethics in Healthcare by Bill Runciman

Books on quality improvement
The classic remains *An Introduction to Quality Assurance* by Avedis Donabedian.
Some books focus solely on healthcare, such as *Quality by Design: A Clinical Microsystem Approach* by Eugene Nelson, Paul Batalden and Marjorie Godfrey.
The majority describe quality improvement and quality assurance in industry, particularly in Japanese industry, and, within that, at Toyota.

---

of the clinician's responsibility to the organisation that employs them, but the latter four, which are inter-related, are completely new. Of these new responsibilities, perhaps the most challenging is the commitment to all people in need, and not just to those people who have been referred.

From one perspective, broken legs do not pose a problem for health services. All the people with broken legs reach the right service,

---

[1] http://astore.amazon.co.uk/betterv-21

Table 1.1 Discharging new responsibilities for improving population health in the 21st century

New responsibility	Action
Value	Getting the right patients to the right resources
Outcomes	Getting the right outcomes for the right patients
Waste	Getting the right outcomes with the least waste
Sustainability	Doing the right things to protect resources for future generations
Equity	Ensuring fairness and justice
Supporting all patients, not just those referred	Creating population-based, integrated systems
Health promotion	Preventing disease and promoting health and well-being

irrespective of the assertiveness of the patient, the patient's social status or the competence and beliefs of a general practitioner. People with cancer also tend to reach the right service, although there may be delays in the time taken to reach the service due to factors relating to the beliefs and behaviours of both patients and clinicians. For people who have one or more long-term conditions, however, many of them who could benefit from the knowledge and skills of specialist services do not because they are not referred (see Figure 1.5). This problem is common for this group of patients.

There are three possible solutions to this problem.

1. Expand the specialist service, but this is rarely possible in an era of constraint.
2. Clarify and implement referral criteria to reduce the size of the problem as depicted in Figure 1.5.
3. Change the way of working in the specialist service such that the knowledge and skills of the specialists can be made available, either directly or indirectly, to all the patients who could benefit (i.e. all those in need), which is likely to be a much larger number than

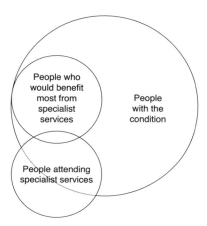

Figure 1.5 The relationship between need and supply

those currently being seen by the specialist service; at present, specialist service resources at present can be accessed only by a patient visiting healthcare real estate.

The changes outlined in point 3 above need to be delivered by clinicians working according to the new paradigm, known as 'population medicine'.

What is different about population medicine?

Population medicine is a style of clinical practice or a way of working. It does not replace other paradigms, such as evidence-based medicine or patient-centred care, but instead it complements and supplements them. When clinicians practising population medicine see individual patients, they continue to use best current evidence and be patient-centred, but they also need to address the root causes of failures in the quality of care. This is best demonstrated by considering the questions clinicians might ask themselves while reflecting on the day's clinic (see Display 1.1). The clinician with a traditional approach asks a different set of questions from that posed by the clinician with a population-medicine perspective, which is based on the 'Five Whys' approach developed by the Toyota Motor Corporation.

Display 1.1 A traditional and a population approach to resolving the problems posed by the presentation of a child with asthma

Scenario: A child with asthma whose problems should have been able to be managed by the child, and the child's family and general practitioner	

Clinician restricted to the traditional responsibilities in healthcare	*Clinician fulfilling the responsibilities of population medicine*
• Why did the child not know how to use her spacer? • Why did the general practitioner refer the child when it would have been possible to resolve the problem using the local clinical guidelines?	• Why was the general practitioner (GP) not able to manage the child without referral? *Because the GP did not follow the guidelines.* • Why did the GP not follow the guidelines? *Because the GP did not know of their existence.* • Why did the GP not know of the existence of the guidelines? *Because the GP was new to the area.* • Why are new GPs not informed about the existence of guidelines? *Because we have no system for identifying and informing new GPs.* • Why do we not set up a process to identify new GPs and pharmacists to ensure they know about local guidelines, resources and referral protocols?

The population medicine approach answers Question 5 by putting in place the necessary systems to prevent a recurrence of the problem.

Another approach using the Five Whys as a foundation would be to ask a different set of questions than the simple rhetorical question, 'Why did the child not know how to use her spacer?' (see Display 1.2). Here are eight questions that a clinician practising population medicine could ask.

Display 1.2 A population approach to the root causes of why children with asthma do not have the knowledge for good self-management

Scenario: A child with asthma who does not know how to use their spacer

1. How many children are there with asthma in the local population?
2. What proportion of children is referred to the specialist service?
3. How many are referred who could be managed by generalists, such as GPs and pharmacists?
4. How many children who should be referred are not?
5. Are we clear about our objectives, guidelines and referral criteria?
6. Are all the generalists working with the local population including those most newly appointed aware of our guidelines and referral criteria?
7. Are all the people with asthma and their carers fully informed about how they can best manage their condition?
8. How good is the service for the local population when compared with services for similar populations in other localities?

From a bureaucratic perspective, the components of a typical health service could be represented as a set of interconnected but separate boxes (see Figure 1.6).

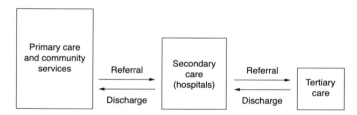

Figure 1.6 The traditional model of institutionalised care

However, there are several mis-representations regarding the depiction of reality in this figure; in reality:

- there are large overlaps between primary and secondary care services, and between secondary and tertiary care services;
- a hospital is portrayed as being different and distinct from 'community' services, but this perpetuates the myth that a hospital is not a community service (1).

11

Another way to depict the relationship of the different types of care is as a Venn diagram (Figure 1.3), in which the different types of care are shown as a set of nested boxes, referred to as 'four-box' healthcare.

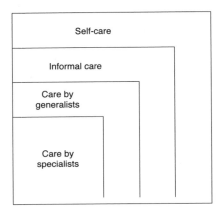

Figure 1.7 'Four-box' healthcare

An individual may make use of all four types of care during the course of a year, or even a day; as can be seen from Figure 1.7, there are 'passages' from one type of care to another. 'Five-box' healthcare is shown in Figure 1.8, revealing the relationship when super-specialist

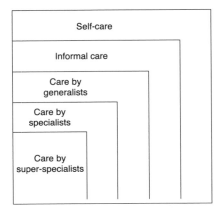

Figure 1.8 'Five-box' healthcare

care (e.g. a paediatric neurology service) is included. The passage from generalist care to specialist care has a filter, as does the passage from specialist care to super-specialist care.

The concept of filters was developed in one of the first books on healthcare systems – *Mental Illness in the Community: Pathways to Psychiatric Care* (4). In this book, several levels of service provision in mental health services were identified together with a filter between each level, as shown Box 1.2. The match between need and resources in mental health services was clearly described and found to be far from perfect.

Box 1.2 Levels of service provision and filters in mental health services (4)

Psychiatrically ill during the year.

FILTER 1: the person's belief about the nature of their problem – e.g. is it normal grief or clinical depression.

Consult their doctor during the year.

FILTER 2: their relationship with their general practitioner and the ease of access.

Recognised as psychiatrically ill by their doctor.

FILTER 3: the generalist's skills.

Referred to a specialist service.

FILTER 4: the generalist's knowledge and beliefs, and the ease of access to the specialist service.

Admitted to a specialist service.

Generalist and specialist partnerships

There is an increasing recognition both implicitly and explicitly that clinicians have responsibilities to the whole population as well as to the individual patient. Although general practitioners have practised population medicine since 1948, when each was allocated a defined population for which they were responsible, and hospital specialists have had some population responsibilities to which they have responded to varying degrees, some recent trends in healthcare management in the NHS, such as the development of Foundation Trusts, have mitigated against the exercise of responsibility for populations.

The relationship between generalists and specialists is often unnecessarily fraught for two reasons.

1. Many members of both types of practitioner fail to understand the difference between the sensitivity of a symptom, sign or test result and its positive predictive value. In general practice, where the incidence and prevalence of disease is lower, the implications of the presence of a symptom, sign or positive test result is of much less concern than in specialist practice where the incidence and prevalence of the disease is much higher, principally because the generalists only refer those patients who obviously have the disease or who have a high probability of having the disease. This leads specialists to criticise generalists for missing 'easy' diagnoses and generalists to criticise specialists for over-investigation.

2. There is an important difference between complex and complicated medical problems. A complex problem is epitomised by an 80-year-old woman with four diagnoses and seven prescriptions, looked after by her 50-year-old daughter who has an alcoholic husband and an unemployed son. This type of situation is standard in general practice. However, when one of the diagnosed diseases becomes complicated, such as heart failure developing in the Parkinson's disease, the generalist seeks specialist help.

To maximise value for the population, it is important:

- To help generalists and specialists work together;
- To recognise the need to use the knowledge and skills of specialists to serve the patients in the population who have not been referred in addition to the patients who have been referred to them;
- To encourage and fund specialists to apply their knowledge and skills to the care of the population in need.

Ways in which value for the population in need can be maximised by hospital specialists working in partnership with generalists are shown in Display 1.3. It is important to emphasise that the specialist or consultant with responsibility for a population does not become

Display 1.3 Specialists and generalists working in partnership to take a population approach to COPD

Scenario: A specialist service for COPD at which 800 patients a year are seen by the consultant in respiratory medicine

- Specialist service to estimate the number of patients with COPD in the population covered by the clinical networks in which the consultant works, based on published epidemiological studies and prescribing data (~2000)
- Conduct an audit across the clinical networks to identify people who have not been referred but who would benefit from referral (~200)
- Hold a joint discussion about how to increase productivity: whether the specialist service should see 1000 extra patients a year using the same level of resources or whether general practitioners manage 200 of the 800 people referred if GPs are given more support by the specialist service
- Specialist service to identify, through an analysis of prescribing and referral patterns, the scope for the specialist service to give greater support to certain general practitioners
- Specialist service to ensure that important new evidence reaches all those healthcare professionals who need to be aware of it
- Specialist service to ensure that all people with COPD receive unbiased information
- Specialist service to accept responsibility for the local variant of the Map of Medicine®
- Specialist service to take responsibility for the professional development of all general practitioners, physiotherapists and pharmacists who are seeing patients with COPD in the population covered by the network
- Specialist service to coordinate and lead the network of all relevant professionals and patient organisations
- Specialist service to produce an annual report

responsible for every patient. The generalist (family doctor, primary care physician or general practitioner) retains responsibility for the patients who are registered with them. Nor does the specialist become responsible for the clinical care of all the individuals in a population. However, they do become responsible for the health of all the people who have the condition about which they have specialist knowledge, and all the people who might develop it (i.e. those who are or could be in need). Thus, they are also responsible not just for the quality and value of care delivered for people with the relevant condition, but also for the prevention of that condition and for helping people with that condition lead a full and healthy life.

To enable clinicians to fulfil all the responsibilities of population medicine:

- these responsibilities need to be recognised in clinicians' job descriptions;
- time should be allocated to enable clinicians to carry out these responsibilities, perhaps one day a week.

However, the lead consultant may also require support for the coordination of the network, with help from a clinical scientist or administrator. A job description with key responsibilities for the clinician who takes the leading role for population medicine is set out in Display 1.4, although it is not envisaged that many clinicians will be full-time in population medicine.

The ethical issues of population medicine

When the topic of population medicine is first raised, some clinicians will be concerned about the potential ethical conflict, as they perceive it, between their total commitment to the individual patient and an explicit responsibility to the population. However, clinicians have always had to manage that most precious of resources, their time, not only by considering what the patient in front of them wants but also the needs of other patients. Although many patients would like more of the clinician's time, all clinicians have to consider how best to use this finite resource.

However, in a situation where clinicians have to make judgements about whether to allocate additional financial resources to the patient in front of them, this does present an ethical problem. The problem can be prevented by ensuring that decisions on the allocation of resources are not made by the individual clinician during a consultation, but through a process that is open and accountable. Daniels and Sabin have expounded the type of accountability necessary for such decision-making.

Accountability for reasonableness is the idea that the reasons or rationales for important limit-setting decisions should be

Display 1.4 Job description for a lead clinician with responsibility for population medicine, taking neurological disease as an example

Aim	• To improve the health of all the people with neurological disease in the local population served
Key result areas	• To promote the prevention of neurological disease • To develop and maintain estimates of the total numbers of people with common neurological disease and problems • For each common neurological disease, to ensure that there is a system of care with appropriate criteria and standards with each system expressed as a care pathway • To build and sustain a clinical network • To work with patients and their representatives to help people with neurological disease to participate as partners in their care and to live a full life and have a good death • To promote research • To produce an annual report for the population served
Resources	The post-holder will have one day a week reserved for this work. They will be supported by an information scientist with knowledge management skills working two days a week and have a small budget to facilitate their work.
Key relationships	• Local branches of relevant patient groups • Local branches of relevant professional associations • Public health professionals serving the population • Relevant managers and policy-makers

publicly available. In addition, these reasons must be ones that 'fair-minded' people can agree are relevant to pursuing appropriate patient care under necessary resource constraints. This is our central thesis, and it needs some explanation.

By 'fair-minded', we do not simply mean our friends or people who just happen to agree with us. We mean people who in principle seek to cooperate with others on terms they can justify to each other. Indeed, fair-minded people accept rules of the game – or sometimes seek rule changes – that promote the game's essential skills and the excitement their use produces. (5)

17

At the beginning of the 21st century, an increasing number of people would agree that it is now unethical not to consider the whole population as well as the individual patient. The principal argument in the debate is about environmental change and resource use, as opposed to lower-value healthcare. These environmental issues, however, are highly relevant and relate to the phenomenon known as 'the tragedy of the commons' in which environmental degradation occurs whenever many individuals use a scarce resource in common (see Display 1.5). Reuben argues that this is the situation in healthcare (6). If every clinician and every patient uses more and more of the finite healthcare resources, there will come a point when the health service breaks down and everyone suffers.

Display 1.5 The tragedy of the commons

Scenario: Imagine you are a farmer grazing your sheep on common land
Custom and tradition mean that you are allowed to have 20 sheep on the common land, but you introduce one more and no-one seems to notice or mind. So the next year you introduce another sheep, and the following year another, and so on. Unfortunately, all the other commoners have adopted the same policy such that a point is reached when the whole ecosystem collapses, the grass does not grow and all the sheep die. This is the tragedy of the commons.

Apart from the danger of service breakdown, in healthcare it is also important to bear in mind that with increasing resource the balance between benefit and harm changes – with increasing resource investment benefit is subject to the law of diminishing returns whereas harm increases in direct proportion to the resources invested; indeed a point may be reached when the increased investment of resources will lead to a reduction in net benefit. Thus, it is important to be cautious about using increased resources, not simply from a financial perspective but also from the perspective of maximising the balance of benefit to harm for the population served.

During the 20th century, healthcare professionals provided health services on the assumption that 'more is better', however, there is a new paradigm for the 21st century:

> *In medicine there are three do's; the can do, the actually do and the should do . . . with the aging of the population and the*

proliferation of the can do, the increase in future healthcare capabilities and costs is an impending tragedy of the commons. The most important challenge for the 21st century is not to expand the can do; rather, it is to bring the care that is provided into line with the should do. Failure to do so will result in a healthcare system that will certainly be fiscally, if not morally, bankrupt. (6)

New skills for population medicine

This book, *How to Practise Population Medicine*, has been prepared to help both the general practitioner consortia involved in commissioning, and hospital and mental health specialists, both medical and non-medical, to develop the knowledge and skills they need for the task of population medicine. It is focused primarily on the new responsibilities of clinicians, and in particular their responsibility to the whole population, not just their responsibility to the proportion of the population in contact with the service. For acute, unequivocal health needs, such as a broken leg, the whole population in need accesses the right service, but this is not the case for many people with chronic health problems.

The focus of management and leadership development in the last decade has been on managing an institution, a health centre or a hospital, although general practitioners have always had a focus on populations. The emphasis on quality improvement, on making care more effective and safer, work that is also focused on institutions, has been essential but is not sufficient to meet the challenges of the 21st century. Practising clinicians today should take responsibility for not just the patients who happen to have made contact with the specialist service but also all the people whose needs could be met, directly or indirectly, by the skills of the specialist service. The skills for population medicine complement and supplement the skills that many clinicians have acquired during the last two decades. Although this new skill set includes general management skills and techniques to improve quality and safety, the skills that clinicians will need to maximise value for the whole population, as well as to improve quality and safety for individual patients, have not hitherto been covered. See Box 1.3.

> **Box 1.3 The skills for population medicine**
> - Maximising value
> - Reducing waste and increasing sustainability
> - Mitigating inequity
> - Promoting health and preventing disease
> - Creating systems
> - Building networks
> - Clarifying pathways
> - Developing budgets
> - Managing knowledge
> - Engaging the population and patients
> - Changing the culture

The need for medical leadership

Of all the skills needed to promote population medicine, that relating to changing the culture might be the most difficult to apply, but culture change is an integral part of leadership. Towards the end of the 20th century, it was accepted that a subset of clinicians had to be given training to develop management skills. Later on, the need to develop leadership skills was also recognised, based on the principle, long accepted in industry, that leadership and management although related required different skill sets: leaders are expected to shape and change culture, whereas managers work within it.

> *When we examine culture and leadership closely, we see that they are two sides of the same coin; neither can really be understood by itself. If one wishes to distinguish leadership from management or administration, one can argue that leadership creates and changes cultures, while management and administration act within a culture.* (7)

Any new culture needs to be inculcated from the first day of professional education. Some medical schools have already recognised the need for a new curriculum to meet the demands and pressures of a world in which there are finite resources, as outlined by Cooke in the *New England Journal of Medicine*:

> *We must ensure that all students acquire a basic understanding of how medical care is financed, where national healthcare policies come from, and the politics that shape financing and workforce choices.* (8)

This task of culture change will not be easy. Clinicians must continue to be committed to the individual patients in front of them, but in the decades to come they will also need to develop a commitment to the whole population, including to the patients they have never seen and may never see.

Questions for reflection or for use in teaching or network building

If using these questions in network building or teaching, put one of the questions to the group and ask them to work in pairs to reflect on the question for three minutes; try to get people who do not know one another to work together. When taking feedback, let each pair make only one point. In the interests of equity, start with the pair on the left-hand side of the room for responses to the first question, then go to the pair on the right-hand side of the room for responses to the second question.

- What are the ethical issues for clinicians whose only concern is for the patients who consult them?
- Although the introduction of free treatment under the NHS in 1948 freed many patients from anxiety about the costs of consulting, what was its effect on the power balance between doctor and patients?
- If we accept that responsibility for quality, equity and ensuring patients are treated with dignity are all essential aspects of good healthcare, are there any other responsibilities in addition to the six listed which clinicians need to fulfil in the 21st century?
- Why should all clinicians be explicitly responsible for these six dimensions or only a proportion of them?

References

(1) Mitton, C. and Donaldson, C. (2004) *Priority setting toolkit. A guide to the use of economics in healthcare decision making.* BMJ Publishing Group (pp. 5–6).

(2) Block, P. (1996) *Stewardship: choosing service over self-interest.* Barrett-Koehler.

(3) Holmgren, D. (2002) *Permaculture.* Holmgren Design Services (p. 5).

(4) Goldberg, D. And Huxley, H. (1980) *Mental Illness in the Community. The Pathway to Psychiatric Care.* Tavistock Publications.

(5) Daniels, N. and Sabin, J. E. (2008) *Setting Limits Fairly, Learning to Share Resources for Health.* Oxford University Press (p. 44).

(6) Reuben, D. (2010) Miracles, choices and justice; the tragedy of the future commons. *JAMA* 304; 467–468.

(7) Schein, E. H. (2004) *Organizational Culture and Leadership.* John Wiley & Sons Inc. (pp. 10–11).

(8) Cooke, M. (2010) Cost consciousness in Patient Care – what is Medical Education's responsibilities? *NEJM* 362: 1253–1254.

2

MAXIMISING VALUE

This chapter will:

- distinguish between the two different types of meaning of value – the moral meaning and the economic meaning;
- give examples of the meaning of the term 'value' when it is used in an economic sense;
- distinguish between quality and value and describe their relationship;
- discuss ways in which the allocation of resources, either between programmes or within a programme, can increase value;
- discuss how the management of innovation and redundancy is essential to maximise value;
- define inappropriate and futile care and how variations in practice may indicate the presence of inappropriate care.

By the end of this chapter, you will have developed an understanding of:

- the difference between the economic meaning of the word value and the moral meaning;
- the relationship between quality improvement and value improvement;
- three types of lower value interventions;
- how those who allocate resources can maximise value, either by the process of allocation or by the way in which they handle innovation and disinvestment;
- how allocation decisions can be made not only between programmes but also within programmes, and even within the budget of resources available for a specific disease;
- the spectrum of care from necessary to futile;

- unwarranted variation and how this should be analysed;
- how variations in the level of health service activity, in particular high rates of intervention, may indicate inappropriate care and the need for patient decision aids.

The end of the quality era

For the last decade, the focus of healthcare managers and clinicians has been on quality improvement. However, as shown in Figure 2.1, focusing on quality alone improves, but does not maximise, value. Value is defined as doing the right things right to the right people.

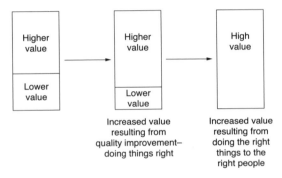

Figure 2.1 Doing the right things right to the right people

There is now a shift in emphasis from quality to value as signalled by an article entitled 'The End of the Quality Improvement Movement: Long Live Improving Value' by Robert Brook, one of the most influential founders of the quality improvement movement.

Instead of trying to fill gaps in knowledge about the epidemiology of quality, the focus should be on developing an epidemiology of value, which contains both measurement of cost and quality, and is applicable to both the developed and the developing world. The results of this work would help to distinguish between a level of quality that is good value and the best available quality that may provide small improvements in health at enormous cost. (1)

As with any paradigm shift, the new paradigm of increasing value embraces and absorbs the older paradigm of improving quality. However, it is necessary to clarify the meaning of the term 'value' in this context.

The meanings of value

For an object, such as a book, it is possible to develop a definition stating what it is; however, for a concept, such as value, it is more productive to identify the various meanings of the term rather than a simple definition.

> *Value in any field must be defined around the customer, not the supplier. . . . Hence it is patient health results that matter, not the volume of services delivered. But results are achieved at some cost. Therefore, the proper objective is the value of health care delivery, or the patient health outcomes relative to the total cost (inputs) of attaining those outcomes. Efficiency, then, is sub-sumed in the concept of value. So are other objectives like safety, which is one aspect of outcome.* (2)

There are many different meanings associated with the word 'value' when used in the context of healthcare.

The moral meaning: 'the status of a thing or the estimate in which it is held according to its real or supposed worth, usefulness, or importance' (a definition from late Middle English in the *Shorter Oxford English Dictionary*). This meaning of the word 'value', often used in the plural, is common in healthcare, for example, the hospital that states 'Our values are to promote patient choice', and 'We respect openness and honesty'. Another term to describe this meaning would be a 'principle'.

The economic meaning: one of the four variants of the term in the *Shorter Oxford English Dictionary* is 'that amount of some commodity, medium of exchange, etc. which is considered to be an equivalent for something else'; an example of the meaning from 1806 which is still relevant two centuries later is given as 'We could hardly be said to have value for our money' (3).

In healthcare, value is measured by the relationship between outcome and cost, as expressed by the following formula:

$$\text{Value} = \frac{\text{Outcomes}}{\text{Costs}}$$

However, because all healthcare can do harm as well as good, the formula needs to be amended to reflect this:

$$\text{Value} = \frac{\text{Good outcomes} - \text{bad outcomes}}{\text{Costs}}$$

As good and bad outcomes are determined by the decisions and actions of professionals, the value of a service depends on:

- whether decision-making is evidence-based;
- the safety of the service;
- the quality of the service.

Thus, the paradigms of high-quality healthcare, evidence-based decision-making and patient safety remain important, but the 21st century is the era of value in which the outcome is the dominant concern.

The meanings of outcome

Following the distinction of outcome from process by Avedis Donabedian, in the early literature on outcome, the most important step was to distinguish process measures from outcome measures. Process measures are easier to define and implement than outcome measures but have less validity. For example, a process measure would be the degree to which a hospital achieved certain safety standards; the outcome measure would be a hospital's standardised mortality ratio (SMR).

However, during the last decade, the focus has shifted to the patient's perception of outcome. Initially, it was thought that patient experience measured service quality with greater validity than patient satisfaction, which is greatly influenced by a patient's expectations. It is now clear that the patient's opinion of the outcome of care must be measured and not simply the patient's experience of the interpersonal aspects of care. Thus, patient-reported outcome measures (PROMs) are seen as outcome measures at least as important as the clinician's perception of the success of an intervention.

The patient's perception of outcome has also become important in the context of an increasing emphasis on the harm of healthcare. In the 20th century, the dominant preoccupation was the benefits of healthcare; in the 21st century, the dominant preoccupation will be the balance between benefit and harm, either from the perspective of the individual patient or from that of the population. In Matrix 2.1, the relationship between benefit and harm from an intervention for individual patients is shown.

Matrix 2.1: Relationship of benefit to harm for individual patients

		Benefits from intervention (good outcome)	
		Present	*Absent*
Harm from intervention (poor outcome)	*Absent*	Very good outcome	Disappointing for the patient: was the decision to intervene correct?
	Present	Perception of outcome dependent on the balance of good and harm and the patient's expectation when consenting (4)	Very bad outcome

To ensure that a high proportion of patients have a good outcome, in addition to making sure that only interventions associated with strong evidence of doing more good than harm are delivered safely and at high quality, the clinician leading a service must take several different approaches:

- To ensure that every patient facing a fateful decision makes it fully informed;
- To ensure that the culture of the clinical service is one in which inappropriate or futile care is discouraged.

Lower-value healthcare

The fact that an intervention is effective, i.e. there is strong evidence that it does more good than harm, does not necessarily mean that it is of high value either to the population or to an individual. The value of an intervention depends on the context in which it is offered, which then determines whether its use is appropriate.

Assessments of the effectiveness of an intervention are objective, whereas assessments of the appropriateness of an intervention are subjective. Clinical judgement is used to place an intervention on the spectrum of appropriateness (see Figure 2.2).

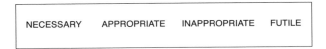

NECESSARY   APPROPRIATE   INAPPROPRIATE   FUTILE

Figure 2.2 The spectrum of appropriateness

There are many definitions of all of the terms on the appropriateness spectrum. However, one of the definitions of a 'necessary' procedure is given in the quotation below:

We define a procedure as necessary – or crucial – if all four of the following criteria are met:

- *The procedure must be appropriate . . .*
- *It would be improper care not to recommend this service.*
- *There is a reasonable chance that the procedure will benefit the patient. Procedures with a low likelihood of benefit but few risks are not considered necessary.*
- *The benefit to the patient is not small. Procedures that provide only minor benefits are not necessary.*

. . . In conclusion, necessity ratings can be used together with appropriateness ratings to address not only the overuse of procedures but also to indicate limited access to care through underuse of procedures. Key words: appropriateness; necessity; crucial; guideline panels. (5)

It is generally accepted that the definition of 'appropriate' in relation to a procedure is that outlined by Kahan et al.:

> *a procedure is termed appropriate if its benefits sufficiently outweigh its risks to make it worth performing, and it does at least as well as the next best available procedure. A procedure is termed inappropriate if the risks outweigh the benefits.* (6)

Although it may be easy to agree upon the general definition of a term such as an 'appropriate' procedure, it is not as easy for a group of doctors to reach agreement when asked to identify whether an intervention is appropriate for a particular patient. Furthermore, it is not easy to reach an agreement on the definition of 'futility' when considered in relation to individual patients, as the following extract from one of the key books on futile intervention shows:

> *Schneiderman and Jecker have suggested that a treatment should be considered futile when it has not worked once in the last 100 times it was tried. Waisel and Truog attack this definition by noting that the criterion is statistically equivalent to saying that a therapy is futile if physicians are 95% confident that it would be successful no more than 3 in 100 – a mathematical truism that Schneiderman et al. had themselves admitted in an earlier publication.* (7)

Clinicians may disagree about what is or is not an appropriate procedure or what is or is not futile care for an individual, but they tend not to be aware that the care offered by their service would be considered inappropriate by other doctors or people in other professional groups.

Two different types of data can highlight the possibility of inappropriate care:

- time trends – as the rate of operation increases, the probability of inappropriate care increases because treatment is offered to people who are less severely affected;
- analysis of variation – high rates of intervention in a population, as revealed by the *Dartmouth Atlas of Health Care* (8) and *The NHS Atlas of Variation in Healthcare* (10), indicate the possibility of unwarranted variation.

More is not necessarily better

Many elective operations are now performed much more frequently than they were in the past. For instance, the rate of cataract operations in England increased significantly from 1989 to 2004 (see Figure 2.3).

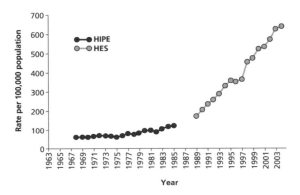

Figure 2.3: Rate of cataract operations per 100,000 population, 1989–2004 (reproduced from the British Journal of Ophthalmology, Tiarnan Keenan, Paul Rosen, David Yeates, Michael Goldacre, Volume 91, pages 901–904 © with permission from *BMJ* Publishing Group Ltd) [Goldacre fig, Atlas 1.0]

Initially, an increase in the number of operations performed represents addressing what everyone would agree was unmet need, such that the increase in the volume of interventions provided is deemed necessary. However, with time, as the absolute number of operations and the rate of intervention increase, people whose need is less severe need receive the intervention, and it is debatable whether the care can be classified as 'necessary'.

Avedis Donabedian was the first to describe what happens as the volume of medical care provided to a population increases and the threshold for intervention changes, originally published in *Explorations In Quality Assessment & Monitoring* (10), but latterly in *Introduction to Quality Assurance in Healthcare* (11). He pointed out that as the amount of resources invested increases, the benefit that results from each unit of increase becomes smaller, known as the law of diminishing returns, whereas the amount of harm done increases in direct proportion to the investment of resources (see Figure 2.4).

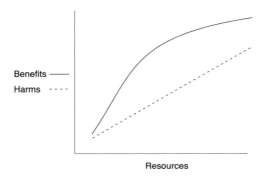

Figure 2.4 The Law of Undiminished Harm

Thus, there is a point when the investment of additional resources will lead to reduction in net benefit or health gain calculated by subtracting the harm from the benefit, as shown in Figure 2.5. The turning point beyond which additional resources do not result in any increase in value Donabedian called the point of optimality.

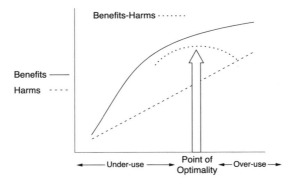

Figure 2.5 The relationship between resources, benefit and harm – under-use, optimality and over-use

Clinicians need to be aware of the point at which the balance between benefit and harm becomes unfavourable. Donabedian described the task as:

The balancing of improvements in health against the cost of such improvements. The definition implies there is a 'best' or

31

'optimum relationship' between costs and benefits of health care, a point below which more benefits could be obtained at costs that are low relative to benefits and above which additional benefits are obtained at costs too large relative to corresponding benefits. (11)

Unknowing and unwarranted variation in practice

The groundbreaking research of Professor John Wennberg at Dartmouth Medical School demonstrated that there were large and unknown variations in clinical practice, such as in the rate of knee operations. Furthermore, much of this variation was not only unknown but also unwarranted, which he defined as:

Variation in the utilization of health care services that cannot be explained by variation in patient illness or patient preferences. (12)

It is important to appreciate that clinicians responsible for providing a greater level of intensity of care were convinced that the level of care was appropriate. No conscientious clinician provides inappropriate care consciously. Every clinician believes that what they deliver is appropriate but, because most clinicians and most local services work in isolation, there is very little awareness of what others do. For this reason, the clinician intervening twice as often as the mean and the clinician intervening half as often as the mean believe they are intervening at the 'right' rate, as does the clinician who intervenes at the mean rate. None of them should necessarily be confident about the level of intervention including the clinician intervening at the mean rate because that may also encompass many inappropriate interventions.

The identification of inappropriate practice can be achieved in several different ways:

- by encouraging clinicians to visit other services or 'buddy' with another service so that exchanges can be arranged – working in another service can be illuminating;
- through peer review of cases and case-notes;
- by identifying and investigating variation in activity – the possi-

bility that there is over-use or under-use of a service is raised if rates of activity are higher or lower than in comparable services caring for similar populations.

The appropriateness of an intervention is distinct from its effectiveness. Appropriateness is determined by the values of the patient. Therefore, it is essential that the patient's values are incorporated into any clinical decision about whether or how to intervene. This can be done by promoting shared decision-making via the use of patient decision aids.

Variations analysis and shared decision-making are both ways in which the 'right' outcomes can be achieved for populations and individual patients, respectively. Furthermore, these methods are inter-related. When rates of intervention are high, the balance of benefit to harm may be beyond the point of optimality from a population perspective. From the perspective of an individual patient, the types of outcome that have to be considered are also different because, as Wennberg highlighted, when there are more resources:

- less severely affected people are being offered interventions;
- for each person, the magnitude of benefit that can be expected is reduced because their problem is less severe to start with, however, the likelihood and magnitude of harm experienced is the same as for more severely affected people.

Wennberg states that if an operation is performed on a patient who does not understand the risks they face, and who would not have accepted the offer of the operation if they had been so informed, the service has operated on 'the wrong patient'.

Seven steps to increase value

Although steps to improve quality and safety lead to better outcomes, there are further steps that a clinician responsible for delivering healthcare to a population can take to increase value in addition to these two core functions of service management (see Box 2.1)

Box 2.1 Seven steps to increase value in healthcare

- Negotiating well with payers and commissioners
- Allocating resources to different patient groups to achieve optimality
- Within each group of patients with the same condition, allocating resources to achieve the optimal balance of prevention, diagnosis, treatment and care
- Ensuring the right patients are seen by the service
- Encouraging innovation and disinvestment to increase value
- Getting the right outcome for the right patient
- Reducing waste (see Chapter 3)

Negotiating well with payers and commissioners

Those who pay for, or commission, healthcare allocate resources to different programme budgets. The allocation of resources in NHS England across 23 programme budget categories is shown in Table 2.1.

One of the key responsibilities for the clinician managing a service is to try to gain additional resources from the organisation that allocates money to all programmes of care. In an era of constraint, this responsibility may become one of trying to prevent the service from suffering cuts.

In times of growth, clinicians managing services have become accustomed to bid for resources to add to the programme budget for their service, relying on the institution allocating resources among programmes to fund in their favour based on the case of need submitted. The case of need, or business case, has traditionally been based on evidence of effectiveness and cost-effectiveness.

Let us take the situation among three programme budgets – respiratory disease, gastro-intestinal disease and cancer – as an example. The respiratory services programme has bid for additional resources. If successful, the respiratory services programme would receive an increased amount of resources and thereby a greater proportion of the budget, whereas the services for people with gastro-intestinal disease and cancer would retain the same absolute

Table 2.1 Programme budgeting estimated England-level gross
expenditure for programmes in 2010/11[1]

Programme budgeting category code	Programme budgeting category	Gross expenditure 2010/11 (£billion)
1	Infectious Diseases	1.80
2	Cancers & Tumours	5.81
3	Disorders of the Blood	1.36
4	Endocrine, Nutritional and Metabolic Problems	3.00
5	Mental Health Disorders	11.91
6	Problems of Learning Disability	2.90
7	Neurological	4.30
8	Problems of Vision	2.14
9	Problems of Hearing	0.45
10	Problems of Circulation	7.72
11	Problems of the Respiratory System	4.43
12	Dental Problems	3.31
13	Problems of the Gastro-Intestinal System	4.43
14	Problems of the Skin	2.13
15	Problems of the Musculo-Skeletal System	5.06
16	Problems due to Trauma and Injuries	3.75
17	Problems of the Genito-Urinary System	4.78
18	Maternity and Reproductive Health	3.44
19	Conditions of Neonates	1.05
20	Adverse Effects and Poisoning	0.96
21	Healthy Individuals	2.15
22	Social Care Needs	4.18
23	Other Areas of Spend/Conditions	25.95
Total		107.00

[1] http://www.dh.gov.uk/health/2012/08/programme-budgeting-data/

amount of resources but receive a smaller proportion of the budget. When making decisions about resource allocation among different programmes of care, decision-makers have to take as a starting position the inherited levels of resource allocation (see Figure 2.6).

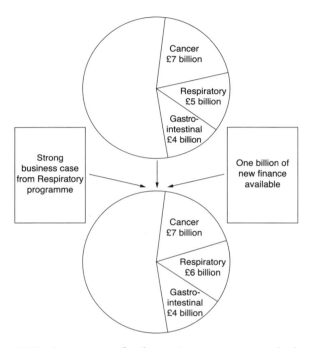

Figure 2.6 Winning resources for the respiratory programme budget when resources are increasing

In times of fiscal constraint when there is no growth in resources, payers and commissioners have to switch resources from one programme budget to another, using a process called marginal analysis.

The task of measuring costs and benefits should be done through marginal analysis. This involves starting with a particular mix of services and analysing changes in that mix. If resources can be shifted to produce greater benefit then this should be done. (13)

The aim is to achieve Pareto optimality, that is, the point at which allocative efficiency is at its maximum when the distribution of resources is such that shifting a pound from one budget to any other would produce no more value. Needless to say, this state of Pareto optimality, analogous to a state of divine grace, has never been reached in any health service. It should be noted that the allocation of resources across programme budget categories in NHS England (Table 2.1) did not necessarily result from a process of logical analysis. It simply represents the end result of decades of ad-hoc decision-making.

In future, the clinician responsible for delivering a service to one subgroup of the population will have to prepare a bid or business case in which it is argued that:

- there is no waste or lower-value activity in their budget;
- if resources were switched from another programme budget, the population as a whole would receive better value (Figure 2.7).

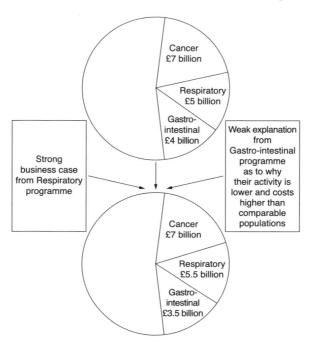

Figure 2.7 Winning resources for the respiratory programme budget when there is no growth in resources

However, before starting marginal analysis, payers and commissioners will expect clinicians to examine their own budgets. Payers and commissioners will want assurance that:

- the entire programme budget is allocated optimally to the different conditions within that programme;
- after allocation the service achieves high value from the resource allocation.

Allocating resources to different patient groups optimally

Unless general practitioners have a special interest in a particular condition or aspect of medicine, as generalists they need to distribute their resources among all their patients as best they can, given that as generalists they deal with all types of health problem. Specialists, however, are frequently faced with more explicit decisions about the allocation of resources among a small number of patient groups or sub-specialties, although specialists also have to take account of patients with rare diseases.

When there are increases in health service investment, the clinician who is a manager bids for more resources to increase the amount invested in the condition for which increased need has been identified – in a sleep apnoea service, for example, where need has increased due to improved diagnosis and the development of new technology. However, when there is no increase in health-service investment, the most likely source of additional finance for sleep apnoea will be from within the respiratory diseases programme budget (see Figure 2.8), which in England is about £100 million per million population.

It is rare that the decision-maker is able to make a decision completely rationally. They must use what Herbert Simon called 'bounded rationality', a principle that the main proponents of systems thinking have adapted and promoted.

> *Bounded rationality arises because human cognitive capabilities, as wonderful as they are, are overwhelmed by the complexity of the systems we are called upon to manage. Chapter 1 discussed bounded rationality; here I repeat Herbert Simon's (Administrative Behaviour, 1957, p. 198) principle of bounded rationality:*

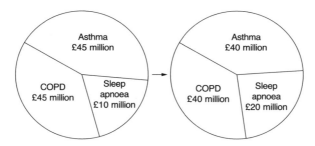

Figure 2.8 Finding resources for sleep apnoea from within the Respiratory Programme Budget (figures are approximations)

'The capacity of the human mind for formulating and solving complex problems is very small compared with the size of the problem whose solution is required for objectively rational behaviour in the real world of even for a reasonable approximation to such objective rationality'. (14)

In making decisions about the care for a population, such as the population of London or a subgroup of the population with common needs such as people with respiratory disease, three factors have to be taken into consideration (see Figure 2.9):

Evidence of good and bad effects of all the interventions;

The value the population places on the benefits and harms of each care option;

The other needs of the population.

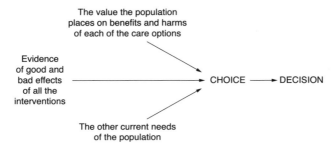

Figure 2.9 Relating the evidence to the needs and values of the population

As the evidence is rarely 100% conclusive and it is impossible to model precisely the impact of the resources used on the whole population, the decision-maker will have to make a value judgement. However, judgement is a subtle concept that has more than one meaning. Furthermore, value judgements often have important ethical elements. Thus, judgement is exercised not only in weighing the different options but also in understanding, calculating and managing the ethical elements of the decision, a complexity that has been described by Herbert Simon.

It is here that judgement enters. In making administrative decisions it is continually necessary to choose factual premises whose truth or falsehood is not definitely known and cannot be determined with certainty with the information and time available for reaching that decision. . . .

In ordinary speech there is often confusion between the element of judgement in decision and the ethical element. This confusion is enhanced by the fact that the further the means-end chain is followed, i.e. the greater the ethical argument, the more doubtful are the steps in the chain, and the greater is the element of judgement involved in determining what means will contribute to what ends. (15)

This exercise of judgement can bring the clinician responsible for the budget into conflict with colleagues, particularly if those colleagues do not feel any responsibility towards the stewardship of resources. In this situation, it can be helpful to provide colleagues with examples of types of activity that can be classified as being of lower value to populations and patients (see Box 2.2).

Achieving optimal balance between prevention, diagnosis, treatment and care for a single group of patients

Value-based decisions also have to be made when considering a single group of patients – people with chronic obstructive pulmonary disease (COPD), for example. The decision to switch resources from domiciliary oxygen to triple therapy could be regarded as one that can be based on evidence of effectiveness because it concerns the

---

Box 2.2 Interventions or services of lower value

- There is clear evidence of ineffectiveness or evidence that they do more harm than good
- There is no or weak evidence of effectiveness but the intervention/service is not being delivered in a context that would enable the collection of evidence to judge effectiveness, e.g. not being delivered as part of an ethically approved, well-designed research project – these interventions are often referred to as 'innovations' or 'developments'
- There is evidence of effectiveness, but the intervention/service is being offered to patients whose characteristics are different from those of the patients in the original research studies that produced the evidence of effectiveness
- They consume resources that would produce more value, i.e. a better balance of benefit to harm, if invested in another intervention/service for the same group of patients

---

best mix of therapies for patients at a particular stage in the course of their disease. However, decision-making about care for a group of patients can include a value judgement because:

the options are rarely directly comparable;

each option may be championed by a colleague who is an enthusiast for their particular intervention, ready to argue why they need more resources or why they should be spared a cut.

This process of achieving an optimal balance in resource allocation for a single group of patients is referred to as 'within-system marginal analysis'. In this type of marginal analysis, the options have to be considered within the limits of the finite resources available for that particular health problem. For instance, the clinician in charge of respiratory services for a population who has already allocated all the resources optimally to the three principal conditions – asthma, sleep apnoea and chronic obstructive pulmonary disease (COPD) – may have to use judgement to decide on the balance of resources between treatment and rehabilitation.

Consider the options facing the clinician responsible for a comprehensive COPD service. They can allocate resources to five different types of intervention – prevention, diagnosis, treatment, rehabilitation and end-of-life or palliative care (see Figure 2.10).

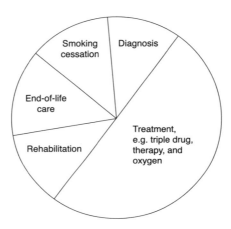

Figure 2.10 Components of the system budget for COPD

To support clinicians in the allocation of resources within a service, tools have been developed by a team at the London School of Economics (LSE) that can enable the value of different choices to be estimated and displayed in order to stimulate discussion and debate.[1] This tool was used by healthcare professionals to assess the relative value of different interventions for COPD. They concluded that:

> *the current sequence of management may need reordering so that interventions such as stop smoking and consideration for referral to pulmonary rehabilitation should happen before any trial of triple therapy.* (16)

The decision to switch resources from treatment to prevention, or vice versa, is a value judgement encompassing ethical elements, as is the decision to switch resources from asthma to COPD or from respiratory disease to cancer.

[1] http://www.health.org.uk/news-and-events/newsletter/star-combining-value-for-money-with-patient-involvement/

Ensuring the right patients are seen

In Chapter 1, it was emphasised that one of the most important actions in population medicine is to ensure that a specialist service sees the right patients, and that the patients being supported by generalists receive the right care. This requires the clinician practising population medicine to be concerned about all the people in the population who have a particular condition, and to support all the clinicians working with that population irrespective of whether those clinicians are generalists or specialists.

Taking a population approach to health services is likely to reduce inequity because there is usually a higher proportion of people from disadvantaged and deprived communities in the subgroup of the population who are either not seen by the specialist service or who do not receive a particular intervention.

Encouraging innovation and disinvestment to maximise value

Another way of classifying the value judgements that a clinician responsible for delivering services to a population has to make is to consider them as investment or disinvestment decisions. Decisions about investment or disinvestment are generated either by the desire to fund an innovation created by either another organisation, such as a new drug or a new piece of equipment, or someone who works in or uses the service (see Figure 2.11).

Encouraging higher-value and discouraging lower-value innovation

Innovation is usually associated with starting new services or procedures. However, two other activities are of greater importance if innovation is to be managed well:

- stopping starting – that is, stopping the drift into practice of lower-value interventions;
- starting stopping – that is, stopping lower-value activities so that resources may be released for re-use, referred to as disinvestment.

Those who manage clinical services have to be alert to the arrival of new technology that does not increase value or, if it does, is introduced before other interventions deemed to be of lower value have been

43

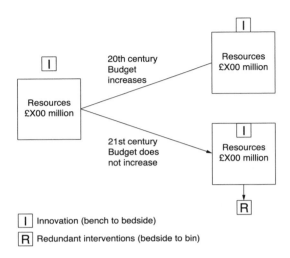

| I | Innovation (bench to bedside) |
| R | Redundant interventions (bedside to bin) |

Figure 2.11 The funding of innovation from disinvestment

stopped or scaled down. Controlling procurement and the order book allows new technology to be appraised, but new technology can bypass appraisal processes in various ways:

- through being lent by the developer;
- by masquerading as research;
- by being given by the manufacturer without an initial charge, or bought by a charity in an attempt to change clinical practice and force the hand of the budget-holder.

Those who manage clinical services must also be alert to the arrival of new knowledge that can increase value. In an ideal world, all clinicians would be motivated not only to adopt new technology but also to monitor new knowledge in order to identify evidence of higher-value interventions, or evidence of ineffective or lower-value interventions which would lead them to start stopping a service or a long-standing clinical practice. However, people tend to be slow to adopt new knowledge even that which does not increase costs – for instance, the evidence that a checklist used before an operation reduces the risk of harm (17). Clinicians may not start stopping long-established practices unless they are motivated to find the resources to fund an innovation that they want and which they believe will add value to the service.

In England, NICE has made a major contribution to improving the management of innovation by the NHS, particularly where new drugs are concerned. New equipment and new procedures, such as new surgical operations or new models of service delivery such as a new screening programme, are more difficult to manage:

- the research to assess their effectiveness is more difficult to undertake;
- implementation is much more difficult, being dependent on the skill of the surgeon or the functioning of a multidisciplinary team, or both.

These difficulties surrounding the management of surgical innovation were addressed in a workshop organised by the Nuffield Department of Surgery, Oxford. This discussion led to a series of articles published in *The Lancet*. The first of the articles described a new paradigm for evaluation of surgical innovation (see Box 2.3).

Box 2.3 A five-stage paradigm for the development of innovative surgical practices (18)

1. Innovation
2. Development
3. Early dispersion and exploration
4. Assessment
5. Long-term implementation and monitoring

In the final article in *The Lancet* series, it was emphasised that the evaluation of new surgical interventions had more in common with the evaluation of complex interventions than it did with pharmacological interventions. This observation led to the proposal of a set of recommendations for the management of surgical innovation (19).

When compared with the management of innovation, it is more difficult to manage the drift to inappropriate and futile care. The phenomenon of drift has been described by David Eddy (20) as being three battles to watch in the 1990s. He highlighted that one of the main factors increasing healthcare costs was 'changes in the volume and intensity' of clinical practice. He argued that this apparently inexorable increase in the volume and intensity of clinical practice must be managed if increasingly scarce resources are to be used effectively.

When an evidence-based innovation is first introduced, it is provided to a group of patients who have characteristics similar to the characteristics of the patients in the original research study in which the evidence base was generated. However, clinicians often have to use their judgement because in clinical practice there are very few patients completely identical to the patients in the original research study. This is because the study design often stipulates entry criteria that are rarely encountered in clinical practice. For instance, the entry criteria for a heart-failure trial might be restricted to people with heart failure under 65 years of age with no co-morbidities, whereas most patients with heart failure are over 65 years of age and have other conditions or co-morbidities. Thus, although clinicians may give the intervention to a tightly defined group of patients to begin with, over the years the intervention may be offered to other patients who have different indications or co-morbidities or who may be less severely affected.

Encouraging disinvestment from lower-value interventions

For the person managing a department or clinical service, there are several approaches to promoting disinvestment in lower-value interventions:

- encouraging innovation within a fixed budget, safe in the knowledge that clinicians will have to do less lower-value work;
- encouraging disinvestment directly, which requires a framework clinicians can use to identify lower-value activities (see Box 2.4).

To maximise value, it is essential to manage both innovation and disinvestment; leaving the maximisation of value to natural evolution is a high-risk strategy unlikely to succeed.

Box 2.4 Framework to identify lower-value activities

- As specialists, are we seeing patients who could be managed equally as well by general practitioners?
- Are there clinical activities for which there is no evidence of benefit that we could stop?
- Are there clinical activities for which there is no supporting evidence that we could stop or have a trial to investigate stopping?
- Can we identify waste, i.e. non-clinical activity that adds no value? (See Chapter 3.)

Getting the right outcome for each individual patient

Changing the traditional view of the 'right' patient outcome

For decades, the definition of 'right' was established by medical opinion until Archie Cochrane published his book *Effectiveness and Efficiency* in 1972 (21). The application of Cochrane's principles to clinical practice was first called 'clinical epidemiology' (22) in a publication of that title written by the team from McMaster University, where so much of the leading work in knowledge management in medicine has been done. From the work at McMaster University, the concept of evidence-based medicine has been developed (18), which emphasises that the making of clinical decisions should be based on best current evidence and not established medical opinion.

> *Evidence-based medicine (EBM) requires the integration of the best research evidence with our clinical expertise and our patient's unique values and circumstances.* (23)

Personalising decisions

The 'right' thing for individual patients is determined by the decisions made by clinicians and patients. For every million population, many decisions are made in the 40,000 consultations that take place daily.

These decisions may be shared between clinicians and patients to a greater or lesser degree during a consultation, but many are taken by either clinicians or patients outside the consultation, such as a patient's decision not to take the medication prescribed for them. The total number of decisions daily is difficult to estimate, but it could be more than 200,000 per million population. These decisions influence both patient outcomes and cost.

Although the development of evidence-based decision-making, supported by services such as NHS Choices and NHS Evidence, has increased the probability of a good outcome, evidence is only one factor in the clinical decision, as illustrated by the simple model of a treatment decision shown in Figure 2.12. From the patient's perspective, the need is for the right intervention, namely, an intervention for which there is a high probability of benefit and a low probability of harm, taking into account the unique clinical condition and values of the patient.

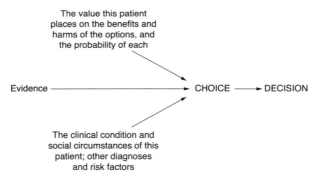

Figure 2.12 Relating the evidence to the needs and values of a particular patient

In the paradigm of evidence-based medicine, the use of best current evidence in decision-making is emphasised, but the clinician needs to relate the evidence, which has often been produced during research studies on patients who are different from the type of patient seen in clinical practice, to the unique clinical needs of each patient. This task can be referred to as personalised medicine.

... two key questions that are most frequently asked by clinicians about applying the results of randomised controlled trials and

systematic reviews to decisions about their individual patients. Is the evidence relevant to my clinical practice? How can I judge whether the probability of benefit from treatment in my current patient is likely to differ substantially from the average probability of benefit reported in the relevant trial or systematic review. (24)

In addition, the development of our understanding of the human genome raises the possibility of using genetic tests to determine which particular treatment option would be best for a particular patient, an activity referred to as precision medicine or stratified medicine.

We define precision medicine as the provision of care for diseases that can be precisely diagnosed, whose causes are understood, and which consequently can be treated with rules-based therapies that are predictably effective.
Another term 'personalized medicine' is often used for this phenomenon that we're calling 'precision medicine'. (25)

Preference-sensitive decisions

The third factor in any decision is the patient's values, that is, what value the patient places on the nature of the good and bad outcomes and on the probabilities of each outcome occurring. In some clinical situations, the issues are clear, such as in the choice of treatment for fractured neck of femur, but in others, such as in the treatment of prostate cancer, the different options for intervention have different consequences. To help patients make the decision best for them, it is essential they are given:

- complete information about the probabilities of good and bad outcomes;
- the opportunity to reflect on how these relate to their values.

The man considering different treatment options for prostate cancer needs support to reflect on whether it is more important for him to avoid incontinence or impotence. Even when the consequences of intervention are less dramatic, in knee replacement for example, the patient needs to reflect on the degree of knee pain and stiffness they are currently experiencing and to consider the possibility that the operation may not be completely successful or could make the pain and stiffness worse. This type of decision has been called a preference-sensitive treatment decision.

> *Preference sensitive treatment decisions involve making value trade-offs between benefits and harms that should depend on informed patient choice.* (26)

In a report for the King's Fund, Mulley et al. have called for an end to the 'silent mis-diagnosis' of patients (27), defined as the failure to diagnose the patient's preferences even though the clinician has diagnosed the disease accurately.

The need for patient decision aids

> *No fateful decision should be made in avoidable ignorance.* (28)

There is now a range of resources to improve decision-making, both for patients and clinicians, many of which were developed by Foundation for Informed Medical Decision Making. The term given to the most structured of these decision-making tools is the patient decision aid.

> *Patient decision aids are designed to support patients in this process; they are intended to supplement rather than replace patient-practitioner interaction. They may be leaflets, interactive media, or video or audio types. Patients may use them to prepare for talking with a clinician, or a clinician may provide them at the time of the visit to facilitate decision making. At a minimum, patient decision aids provide information about the options and their associated relevant outcomes.* (29)

To support patients and clinicians during shared decision-making, patient decision aids have been developed in recognition of the constraints that time places on face-to-face consultations. The consultation remains crucial because clinical judgement has an important part to play in identifying the patient's preferred style of decision-making; many patients still want their clinician to make the decision. However, the consultation can be supplemented and complemented by decision aids.

There is now an extensive and strong evidence base about the problems patients face in making the choice that is right for them, and a growing evidence base about the steps that can be taken to improve a patient's decision-making (see Box 2.5). The steps to improve decision-making need to be managed as actively as the processes involved in the management of safety by the clinician responsible for a service.

Box 2.5 Steps that can be taken to improve decision-making (30)

- Presenting evidence about benefit or harm in relative terms rather than absolute terms results in the patients, and doctors, choosing different options; the use of absolute numbers, such as the number needed to treat (NNT), is more easily under-stood than presenting them in relative terms, such as relative risk Recognising that the research literature has a positive bias thereby giving the impression of greater benefit than is the case
- Offering all patient full information about the options because it is not possible to predict how much information a patient will want on the basis of their age or educational attainment – giving full information in a way that suits the needs of individual patients will not increase the demand for resources; indeed, evidence shows that it can decrease demand (27)
- Identifying patients' preferences for style of decision-making – not all patients like the same style: some prefer to take the lead, some prefer the clinician to take the lead, and some prefer shared decision-making (31)
- Improving clinicians' skills in identifying the patient's pre-ferred style of decision-making: many clinicians cannot discern which style of decision-making an individual patient prefers
- Using patient decision aids to help the patient weigh up the values they place on the benefits and the harms, and the probabilities of each outcome and to overcome the constraints of time in face-to-face decision-making

---

However, it is clear that many fateful decisions are still made in 'avoidable ignorance'. Some of these fateful decisions concern elective surgery, others are about cancer treatment, and many are about end-of-life care. Indeed, the importance of distinguishing effectiveness and quality from outcome is particularly pertinent during end-of-life care. Many people receive effective, high-quality interventions when the outcome they most desire is a good death in their own home.

It is not possible to maximise value for a service and for a population without maximising the value for each individual patient.

Questions for reflection or for use in teaching or network building

If using these questions in network building or teaching, put one of the questions to the group and ask them to work in pairs to reflect on the question for three minutes; try to get people who do not know one another to work together. When taking feedback, let each pair make only one point. In the interests of equity, start with the pair on the left-hand side of the room for responses to the first question, then go to the pair on the right-hand side of the room for responses to the second question.

- What is the best way to explain value to members of the public meeting to consider the budget of a health service?
- When looking for greater value, should the focus be on marginal analysis or on the main budget for a programme?
- How can clinicians be best encouraged to disinvest?
- In what way can patient decision aids help an individual patient make the decision that is right for them?
- What are the responsibilities for the clinician when ensuring that patients make the decision that is right for them?
- What steps could be taken to reduce inappropriate and futile care?

References

(1) Brook, R. H. (2010) The End of the Quality Improvement Movement: Long Live Improving Value. *JAMA*, 304: 1832.

(2) Porter M. E. (2008) What is Value in Health Care? Harvard Business School. Institute for Strategy and Competitiveness. White Paper.

(3) Gray, J. A. M. (2007) *Better Value Healthcare.* Offox Press.

(4) Gigerenzer, G. and Edwards, A. (2003) Simple tools for understanding risks from innumeracy to insight. *Brit. Med. J.* 327: 741–4.

(5) Gray, J. A. M. (2005) *The Resourceful Patient.* Offox Press.

(6) Kahan, J. P. et al. (1994) Measuring the necessity of medical procedures. *Med. Care* 32: 352–365.

(7) Schneiderman, L. J. and Jecker, N. S. (1995) *Wrong Medicine: Doctors, patients and futile treatments.* Baltimore: Johns Hopkins University Press.

(8) Dartmouth Atlas

(9) Right Care (2010) *The NHS Atlas of Variation in Healthcare. Reducing unwarranted variation to increase value and improve quality.* NHS. http://www.rightcare.nhs.uk/atlas/

(10) Donabedian, A. ()

(11) Donabedian, A. (2002) *An Introduction to Quality Assurance in Health Care.* Oxford University Press.

(12) Wennberg, J. E. (2010) *Tracking Medicine.* Oxford University Press.

(13) Mitton, C. and Donaldson, C. (2004) *Priority setting toolkit. A guide to the use of economics in healthcare decision making.* BMJ Publishing Group. (p. 18)

(14) Sterman, J. D. (2000) In: *Business Dynamics: Systems Thinking and Modeling for a Complex World.* The McGraw-Hill companies Inc. p. 598.

(15) Simon, H. A. (1997) *Administrative Behaviour. A study of decision-making processes in administrative organizations.* (Fourth edition). The Free Press. (p. 60).

(16) Gray, J. A. M. and El Turabi, A. (2012) Optimising the Value of Interventions for Populations. *British Medical Journal* doi 10.1136/bmje6192

(17) Gawande, A. (2003) *Complications: A Surgeon's Notes on an Imperfect Science.* Profile Books Ltd.

(18) Barkum , J. S. et al. (2009) Evaluation and stages of surgical innovation. Surgical Innovation and Evaluation, 1. *Lancet* 374: 1089–96.

(19) McCulloch, P. A. and Schuller, F. (2010) Innovation or regulation? The IDEAL opportunity for consensus. *Lancet* 376: 1034–5.

(20) Eddy, D. M. (1993) Three battles to watch in the 1990s. *JAMA* 270: 520–526.

(21) Cochrane, A. (1972) *Effectiveness and Efficiency.*

(22) Haynes, R. B., Sackett, D. L., Guyatt, G. H. and Tugwell, P. (2004)

Clinical Epidemiology: How to Do Clinical Practice Research. Third edition. Lippincott Williams and Wilkins.

(23) Straus, S. E., Richardson, W. S., Glasziou, P. and Haynes, R. B. (2005) *Evidence-Based Medicine. How to practice and teach EBM.*(3rd Edition). Elsevier Churchill Livingstone (p. 1).

(24) Rothwell, P. M. (2007) The *Lancet.* Treating Individuals: from randomised trials to personalised medicine. Oxford: Elsevier Limited.

(25) Christensen, C. M., Grossman, J. H. and Hwang, J. (2009) *The Innovator's Prescription. A Disruptive Solution for Health Care.* McGraw-Hill Professional.

(26) Christensen, C. M. (2003) *The Innovator's Dilemma.* Harper Business Essentials.

(27) Mulley, A., Trimble, C. and Elwyn, G. (2012) *Patients' Preferences Matter: Stop the Silent Misdiagnosis.* King's Fund, London.

(28) Mulley, A., personal communication.

(29) Elwyn, G. (2006) Developing a quality criteria framework for patient decision aids; online international Delphi Consensus process.*BMJ*, 333: 17–427.

(30) O'Connor, A. M. et al. (2007) Toward the 'Tipping Point': Decision aids and informed patient choice. *Health Affairs* 26: 716–725.

(31) Gigerenzer, G. and Gray, J. A. M. (2010) *Better Doctors, Better Patients, Better Decisions.* MIT Press.

3

REDUCING WASTE AND INCREASING SUSTAINABILITY

This chapter will:
- discuss the principal steps that can be taken to reduce the cost of healthcare;
- explain *muda* and its relevance to healthcare;
- provide a classification of different types of waste in healthcare;
- give a definition of sustainability;
- summarise the carbon reduction policy and plan for the NHS;
- outline the contribution of clinical practice to the carbon footprint of the NHS;
- summarise the key characteristics of low-carbon clinical practice.

By the end of the chapter, you will have developed an understanding of:
- the three steps that can be taken in health services to reduce cost;
- the Toyota seven-step approach to the reduction of waste, and how it has been adapted for healthcare;
- the meaning of cost-effectiveness analysis;
- the meaning of the term 'sustainable development';
- the way in which clinical teams can be motivated to take action on sustainability within a health service;
- the strategy that needs to be adopted to reduce the carbon footprint of clinical practice.

Responsibility for reducing waste and increasing sustainability

As discussed in Chapter 2, value is determined by the relationship between outcome and the resources used. It is the responsibility of the clinician serving a particular population to minimise the amount of resources used. Minimising resource use contributes to increasing sustainability. In the context of sustainability, the use of the term resources does not refer to money alone.

The relationship between reducing waste and increasing sustainability is shown in Figure 3.1. The reduction of waste in health services has immediate benefits because it can release resources which are then available to treat more members of the population. However, there are other longer-term benefits that result not only from reducing waste in healthcare but also from increasing the level of sustainability.

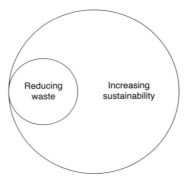

Figure 3.1 The relationship between waste and sustainability

To be a good steward of resources for the population, clinicians practising population medicine need to reduce waste and increase sustainability, and not simply to cut budgets. Clinicians must prevent the waste of time, the time of both clinicians and patients, and the unnecessary use of carbon.

Down with *muda*

In the absence of new resources, those who manage healthcare, most of whom are clinicians, must obtain greater value from the resources available in order to meet increasing need and demand. One way to obtain greater value is to reduce waste. In this situation, there is much to learn from Toyota's success, which is due to an obsession with:

- *kaizan*, the relentless pursuit of better quality, and mass customisation, the analogue of personalised medicine;
- the eradication of *muda*, or waste, which Toyota define as ' . . . *any activity, service, or supply that consumes time, money, and other resources, but creates no value.*' (1)

The Toyota formula, which can be applied to health services (2), is:

Work done = Work that produces value + Waste

It was Taiichi Ohno, one of the driving forces behind Toyota, who created the obsession with *muda* or waste. He identified seven categories of waste in industrial systems, which are relevant to healthcare:

1. Overproduction;
2. Time on hand (waiting);
3. Stock on hand (inventory);
4. Waste of movement;
5. Defective products;
6. Transportation;
7. Processing.

Ohno's work, and the concept of 'lean thinking' (3) which flowed from it, are of central importance to those who pay for, or manage, health services. Indeed, Ohno's seven categories of waste have been adapted and expanded in a book by Toussaint, Gerard and Womack (4), specifically aimed at healthcare professionals (see Box 3.1).

The magnitude of waste is huge. In an impotant article, Don Berwick estimated that the cost of waste 'exceeds 20% of total health care expenditure' (5). The six types of waste he identified are:

- Overtreatment;

Box 3.1 Eight types of waste in healthcare (4)

- Defect: making errors, inspecting work already done for error;
- Waiting: for test results to be delivered, for an appointment, for a bed, for a release of paperwork;
- Motion: searching for supplies, fetching drugs from another room, looking for proper forms;
- Transportation: taking patients through miles of corridors, from one test to the next unnecessarily, transferring patients to new rooms or units, carrying trays of tools between rooms;
- Overproduction: excessive diagnostic testing, unnecessary treatment;
- Overprocessing: a patient being asked the same question three times, unnecessary forms, nurses writing everything in a chartinstead of noting exceptions;
- Inventory: too much or too little; overstocked drugs expiring on the shelf, under-stocked surgical supplies delaying procedures while staff go in search of needed items
- Talent: failing to listen to employee ideas for innovation

- Failures of care co-ordination;
- Failures in execution of care processes;
- Administrative complexity;
- Pricing failures;
- Fraud and abuse.

High-value healthcare involves getting the right patients to the right service and the right treatment done right first time. When taking decisions about what is 'right', lower-value activities need to be identified and excluded. It is also essential to identify and reduce waste, even when the right interventions are being delivered safely and at high quality to the right patients.

Clinicians responsible for serving a population need to minimise waste for two main reasons:

- they have a responsibility to the population providing the resources for healthcare not to waste those resources, which could otherwise be spent on other public services such as education or social services;

- to release resources so that more people in the population can be treated.

Eight questions to help clinicians identify and minimise waste are shown in Box 3.2.

Box 3.2 Questions to identify waste in health services (4)

Can we make more use of buildings and equipment?
Do we need to carry as much stock?
Can the numbers of non-clinical staff be reduced?
Can the waste of clinician and patient time be reduced?
Is care being delivered in the right place?
Could care be provided by less highly paid staff?
Can we use cheaper drugs and equipment?
Can we prevent waste of human resources?

Question 1: Can we make more use of buildings and equipment?

In most countries, hospitals serve small populations of 100,000–300,000 people. This pattern of development was initiated in an era in when:

- there was little specialisation other than that between medical and surgical specialties;
- car ownership was low;
- medical technology, such as imaging technology, was much simpler and less expensive than it is today;
- the mobile 'phone had not even been imagined.

Today, we have a configuration of health services in which there are too many hospitals with under-utilised buildings and equipment. The considerable growth in the size of hospitals during the last 50 years has largely been characterised by development in isolation and development in competition – the 'medical arms race' – 'St Elsewhere's has just bought a CT scanner; we have to have one too.' Not every hospital needs to provide every specialty and every piece of equipment. For hospitals to give up a specialty or to choose not to develop a specialty requires strong clinical leadership. Clinicians practising population medicine to be able to justify and explain that it is in the best interests of the population served, to whom they are accountable, for some members of that population to have to travel further for certain services such that resources are not used in the unnecessary duplication of services. Saving the resources entailed in duplication will enable a greater number of patients to be treated; fortunately, this strategy is also often in the best interests of the individual patient.

Question 2: Do we need to carry as much stock?

> In 2005, 574 different head and socket combinations were used in [hip replacement] operations in England and Wales. It seems implausible that meaningful data can be gathered, or that money can be saved through bulk purchase, when such a number of products and supplies is used in this way. (6)

Just-in-time delivery of the equipment needed was one of the great achievements of the Toyota production systems, and provides much useful learning for health services. In contrast, most health services buy too much equipment of too many types and store it for too long.

Such waste can be prevented partly by improving procurement practices, but staff responsible for procurement do not act in isolation. They tend to buy what clinicians want, seeking the lowest possible price but not necessarily questioning the added value of the new item that a clinician has requested. Indeed, the rigorous appraisal of requests relating to clinical procurement must be done by the clinician leading on population medicine, who needs to persuade colleagues that it is not only the cost of new medical devices that wastes resources but also the costs of storage, stock control and the disposal of unused or unwanted devices. Pharmacies represent a model of good stock control that other hospital departments can follow.

Question 3: Can the numbers of non-clinical staff be reduced?

Contrary to popular belief, administrative staff do not create their own work.

- The work of staff in the central management of a health service is created by outside agencies, which impose certain tasks or require specific information on a regular basis.
- Much of the work of administrative staff in clinical areas is created by clinicians; some of the administrative tasks may be unnecessary tasks but only because clinicians have not addressed the need to make the work of 'clinical microsystems' leaner.

> *A clinical microsystem is a small group of people who work together on a regular basis to provide care to discrete subpopulations of patients. It has clinical and business aims, linked processes, and a shared information environment, and it produces performance outcomes. Microsystems evolve over time and are often embedded in larger organizations. They are complex adaptive systems, and as such they must do the primary work associated with core aims, meet the needs of their members, and maintain themselves over time as clinical units.* (7)

Even teams that work well together may undertake lower-value activities that have crept into their clinical practice over the years, and which need to be eradicated, such as:

- collecting data which no-one uses;
- handovers done on paper that could be done digitally;
- failing to involve the patient as a key member of the team.

Question 4: Can the waste of clinician and patient time be reduced?

For clinicians, time is the scarcest resource: it is finite and once expended cannot be recovered. Unfortunately, much of a clinician's time is wasted. Often, the job of a clinician involves more than encounters with patients during clinical practice. It can encompass management, education and research, and all aspects of a clinician's job, including clinical practice can incur a waste of time.

Waste of time in management

Many physicians are reimbursed for half a day to recognise the time spent in managing resources, but much of this can be considered a "waste", undertaking activities such as:

- writing a plan that has no possibility of realisation;
- contributing to projects that are poorly managed or do not deliver the anticipated outputs;
- meetings without purpose or conclusion.

All clinicians are more than likely to have their own ideas about what constitutes a waste of time, but their perceptions may not be shared. Attendance at a management meeting may be considered a waste of time by a clinician, but regarded as high value by a manager. Independent evaluation is required to determine which of the two perceptions is correct: the clinician because the meeting was unfocused and unproductive, or the manager because the clinician came to a meeting that was of value but with the wrong attitude.

Waste of time in education

Education can have benefits, but it is always associated with a cost. Education is of low value or represents a waste of time if:

- the intervention has been selected in accordance with the clinician's desire rather than through a formal assessment of learning needs – there is evidence that if clinicians are interested in a topic, they will seek the learning they need (8); expenditure on formal training should be reserved only for areas of clinical practice in which the clinician needs to improve the quality of care being delivered or as part of a planned innovation;
- the educational methods employed are not supported by evidence of effectiveness; lectures are usually of low value.

Waste of time in research

The value of investing public money in research is hotly debated, but most countries in Europe and North America now realise that it is important to develop an economy based on knowledge rather than one based on exporting agricultural products or manufactured goods.

Once the funding agency has allocated the financial resources to the clinical researcher, there is much that could be done to increase the level of productivity in research (9). Chalmers and Glasziou identified waste at all four stages of the research process (see Box 3.3).

Box 3.3 Avoidable waste in the clinical research process (9)

- Choosing the wrong question for research
- Doing studies that are unnecessary or poorly designed
- Failing to publish results promptly or not at all
- Producing biased or unusable reports of research

Chalmers and Glasziou concluded that:

> . . . *action to address this waste is needed now because it has human as well as economic consequences.* (9)

Waste of time in clinical practice

Clinical practice is of high value, but within the course of clinical work the time of clinicians is wasted if:

- the patient's notes are missing;
- key data, such as laboratory results, are not available;
- there is unnecessary waiting time, such as between operations in theatre.

Wasting the time of patients

The problems that incur a waste the time for clinicians can also waste the time of patients, especially as there is increasing recognition that patients have to make a significant contribution to their own care even if they do not have to pay for the cost of it. The concept of a 'treatment burden' draws attention to the four types of 'work' that patients with complex problems have to undertake (see Box 3.4). Considering the burden of work for patients receiving care, it is important that clinicians and other healthcare professionals give careful consideration to the ways in which patients' time is wasted and how this may be ameliorated.

Box 3.4 Work undertaken by patients with complex problems during treatment (10)

- Learning About Treatments and Their Consequences: Sense-making Work
- Engaging with Others/Mobilizing Resources: Participation Work
- Adhering to Treatments and Lifestyle Changes: Enacting Work
- Monitoring the Treatments: Appraisal Work

Question 5: Is care being delivered in the right place?

Many patients receive care at healthcare facilities where the levels of staffing and other resources are of an intensity unnecessary for good patient outcomes. Examples of patients usually cared for in secondary care facility who could be cared for elsewhere are given below.

- Patients, usually older people, who have recovered from the acute phase of their disease but cannot be discharged because they are too disabled to return home and yet cannot be found a place in a nursing home. This situation is of concern not only for those who manage or pay for care but also for the patients who are at high risk of hospital-acquired infection, institutionalisation, and malnutrition.
- Patients who attend a clinic with a problem that could have been resolved if their primary care clinician had had a convenient and fast method of accessing the expertise of the specialist, such as via an email, a 'phone call or a video link.

People who die in hospital who could have been supported to die at home.

Question 6: Could care be provided by less highly paid staff?

Highly trained staff are scarce and expensive to train. It is a waste of skill if highly trained staff undertake tasks that could be managed equally well by other staff who have not had the same level of training but whose training has enabled them to carry out a specific range of tasks. Less highly trained staff are able to undertake repetitive tasks with greater attention to detail and to obtain better results than those achieved by the most highly trained staff for whom such tasks are not relevant to their core function.

Question 7: Can we use cheaper equipment and drugs?

The key question when considering waste in relation to equipment and drugs is why pay more than is necessary? Costs can be reduced by:

- skilful procurement;
- bulk purchase;
- the use of generic rather than branded drugs;
- 'making' rather than 'buying';
- sharing services.

These activities are ethically important because they reduce waste, increase productivity and release resources for clinical care. In a significant policy commitment in the White Paper, *Equity and Excellence: Liberating the NHS* (11), the Government stated that '*we will pay drug companies according to the value of new medicines*', a policy referred to as value-based pricing. (12)

Moreover, there are often alternatives to interventions, and the clinician can choose the one that is more cost-effective. The aim of cost-effectiveness analysis is to identify the lowest cost option.

> ... *[cost-effectiveness analysis] compares the costs of alternative ways of achieving a given objective. Where two or more interventions are found to achieve the same level of benefits, the intervention with the least cost is the most cost-effective alternative.* (13)

> *Cost-effectiveness analysis (CEA) is used to address questions of technical efficiency. It is applied in situations where a choice between at least two options with the same goal must be made. That is, given that a particular goal is to be achieved for a fixed budget, CEA can provide a response to the question, 'What is the best way to obtain that goal?* (14)

Once cost-benefit or cost-utility analysis has been used to assess whether an intervention offers good value, cost-effectiveness analysis allows the comparison of two or more methods of achieving the result.

- If cost-benefit analysis demonstrates the value of revascularisation of the coronary arteries, cost-effectiveness analysis enables two methods, coronary artery bypass grafting and stenting, to be compared.
- If cost-benefit analysis demonstrates that the treatment of less severe depression appears to have benefit, cost-effectiveness analysis can be used to answer the question of whether it is less costly to use drugs or cognitive therapy.

Irrespective of the answer to questions posed during cost-effectiveness analysis, there is a supplementary question concerning costliness, for example:

- Which drug is the least costly?
- Is face-to-face or online consultation less costly?

Such questions are often more subtle and less clear-cut than would appear at first sight. There may be small differences in the magnitude of the benefits and harms of each option, or in the probabilities of good and bad outcomes. The decisions about which of the options to choose involve not only a cost comparison but also a judgement about which of the trade-offs associated with each option is preferred in the current context. The simplest type of comparison is that regarding the use of a generic drug when compared with the proprietary product because both interventions are identical in effect but different in price. However, there is evidence that many clinicians do not choose the cheapest option in this situation.

Question 8: Can we prevent waste of human resources?

Demanding though it may be to work on the Toyota production line, that task is much simpler than those associated with clinical practice. For many people, the admonition not to waste the untapped potential of professionals would be interpreted as a call to provide more and better quality continuing professional development. However, greater challenges face the clinician responsible for delivering a service to a population:

- staff retention and turnover – investment in training does not realise much value if a high proportion of those trained, such as nurses, leave within five years;
- burnout – the largest waste of professional talent, particularly when considering the case of clinicians.

> *Burnout is usually identified by three major symptoms: emotional exhaustion, depersonalisation, and decreased sense of self-efficacy. But burnout, we believe is also a euphemism for what many physicians experience as a crisis of meaning and identity. Burnout is the index of dislocation between what people are and what they have to do. It represents an erosion in values, dignity, spirit, and will – and erosion of the human soul.* (15)

The main concern about burnout is not necessarily the loss of workforce and the waste of resources involved in workforce training, but that healthcare professionals can begin to work in a way that is detrimental to the service, annoying for colleagues and upsetting for any patients they may encounter. As pressure increases to meet rising need and demand in a context of no new resources while also continuing to improve quality and safety, in the absence of good leadership, the prevalence of burnout will increase. Indeed, the prevalence of burnout may be worsened by the need for managers to impose what has been called the target culture. The impact of burnout in the United States of America could be serious, especially in the context of implementing universal coverage, but it is by no means a problem unique to the USA.

> *For reform to achieve its goal of providing all residents access to high quality medical care, efforts to identify and address the controllable factors contributing to burnout among physicians are needed.* (16)

Even when burnout is not a problem experienced by physicians and other healthcare professionals, staff can behave in other ways that are counter-productive and difficult to deal with such as the subtle withdrawal of enthusiasm. In developing a health service for a population, it is essential not only to be concerned about strategy and systems, but also to consider and empathise with the situation of frontline staff. The words of Viscount Slim, perhaps Britain's most respected leader in the Second World War, are resonant here. He recognised the need to support personnel in a way that enables them to apply their character traits to the fulfilment of their responsibilities:

> . . . *the high quality of the individual soldier, his morale, toughness and discipline, his acceptance of hardship and his ability to move on his own feet and to look after himself.* (17)

Reducing waste contributes to increased sustainability

Sustainability is a key concept for the 21st century, and the reduction of waste increases the sustainability of any organisation. However, sustainability covers a much broader range of topics than the reduction of waste, and it is of central importance to population medicine, although healthcare in general needs to become much more sustainable (18).

Although the waste reduction is important, it is not sufficient when identifying ways in which to increase sustainability (and value). The clinician fulfilling responsibilities for population medicine needs to consider the impact of clinical practice on the environment and not just the amount of resources consumed. In the UK, the renal service has set the standard for establishing sustainability as a central concern in clinical practice (19). The change in culture necessary to make sustainability a central concern, and not one at the margins, is one of the most important responsibilities in population medicine. Clinicians who manage healthcare need:

- to reduce the carbon footprint of their services;
- to increase the sustainability of their services.

Just as more of the same is not the way to meet the challenges of the future, neither is less of the same.

The meaning of 'sustainable development'

Sustainable development has been described as 'protecting resources from one generation to the next' (20). However, the term 'sustainable development' is widely used and has different meanings for different people. Originally, the term was taken to have an environmental meaning, such as that shown in Box 3.5.

Box 3.5 The environmental meaning of sustainable development (21)

- Consuming fewer material goods
- Using locally produced goods and services to reduce their carbon emissions from their transportation – this will also contribute to the economic sustainability of local communities
- Ensuring that goods and services are produced in as energy-efficient a way as possible with minimal waste (which is recycled)
- Ensuring material goods (such as washing machines, TVs, fridges, etc.) are themselves energy efficient

---

The term, however, now has a broader meaning, perhaps best expressed in the following quotation from *The Lancet*'s Global Health Commission:

> *The concept of sustainable development was formulated to address issues of intergenerational equity in resource availability. It has been condemned as lacking definition and conceptual rigour. However, it offers the possibility of fundamental changes to the way we consume and produce, the way we arrange our functionally fragmented institutions, and the way we distribute resources globally and locally. Most importantly, sustainable development not only posits environmental degradation and poverty as interconnected issues, but it gives an example of how mainstream politics might be brought into a debate that demands a complete rethink of our institutions, resources, and environmental outcome, and also assumes that thee issues can be solved with political will.* (22)

Although sustainability now encompasses many issues, carbon and its effect on climate change are of vital concern to healthcare professionals given that climate change is one of the principal threats to global health in the 21st century. This may be the reason why this issue tends to have the greatest potential for motivating frontline staff. Thus, implementing a concern for sustainability can be encapsulated within a carbon reduction strategy. The NHS Carbon Reduction Strategy for England was first published in 2009. Eight key areas for action were identified, including energy and carbon management.

> ... *NHS scenarios in a low carbon world need to be developed to understand the different ways healthcare delivery must be shaped for a low carbon future. The impact this will have on models of care, and how to develop and promote low carbon pathways, must be understood.*
>
> *This strategy sets the ambition for the NHS to play a leading and innovative role in ensuring the shift to a low carbon society.* (18)

The NHS Sustainable Development Unit (SDU) produces a range of materials for staff, highlighting the short- and long-term benefits of carbon reduction. It emphasises that the NHS must meet the targets enshrined in the Climate Change Act 2008 (see Box 3.6), but by so doing many health and financial co-benefits will also be realised.

Box 3.6 Carbon reduction targets for NHS England (on a 1990 baseline) (23)

- A reduction of 34% by 2020
- A reduction of 64% by 2030
- A reduction of 80% by 2050

Reducing the carbon footprint of healthcare

In Chapter 2, the drive to increase value was described in terms of being able to release resources – whether those resources are time, staff or money – for reallocation to meet some other need. However, this presupposes that the only relevant currency is money, whereas another important currency is carbon.

The NHS, as for all other organisations both public and private, needs to reduce its carbon footprint. The NHS is the largest public sector contributor to climate change through its carbon emissions (18) – 21 million tonnes of CO2 equivalents (MtCO2e) in 2007. (23) The main sources contributing to NHS England's carbon footprint are shown in Figure 3.2.

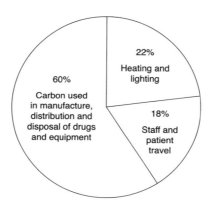

Figure 3.2 Sources contributing to the carbon footprint of NHS England (18)

Although the energy used in heating and lighting the buildings of a health service is considerable and responsible for one-fifth of the carbon footprint, it is not the largest contributor. Three-fifths of the NHS' carbon footprint can be attributed to the manufacture, distribution, use and disposal of drugs and equipment, the "tools" of clinical research and practice. Thus, even if every hospital and health centre converted to renewable energy, the NHS would not achieve its challenging targets for carbon reduction (see Box 3.6). Despite the fact that it is important to reduce the energy use of healthcare buildings:

- it is vital to reduce the amount of carbon used during clinical research and practice;
- it is necessary to reduce the carbon used during staff and patient travel – this contributes almost as much to the carbon footprint as heating and lighting.

This is why the emphasis in the White Paper *Equity and Excellence: Liberating the NHS* (11) on reducing the NHS' carbon footprint is not limited to health services using less energy, it also requires clinicians to change the way in which they deliver care.

Carbon will become an increasingly important constraint in the planning and delivery of health services. Already in the UK, hospitals have been given carbon budgets. These budgets will not grow, even if more money should become available; instead carbon budgets will decrease year on year in order to meet the targets set in the NHS England Carbon Reduction Strategy (see Box 3.6).

Unusually for preventive interventions, the payback time for some carbon reduction measures is rapid. In the White Paper, it is anticipated that cash can be released within the same year by 'improving energy efficiency and developing more sustainable forms of delivery' (11).

Sustainable clinical practice

To reduce the NHS' carbon footprint substantially requires a change in the style of clinical practice. Frances Mortimer, Medical Director of the Centre for Sustainable Healthcare, has developed a model of sustainable clinical practice (see Box 3.7).

Box 3.7 Model of sustainable clinical practice (24)

- All clinicians should be involved in prevention, the most sustainable type of health service
- Patient-centred care, for example, sending most laboratory results directly to patients to reduce the number of trips to health centres to collect results
- Leaner pathways, reducing the number of outpatient and follow-up appointments of low or no value
- The consideration of carbon costs as well as financial costs when considering the cost-effectiveness of treatment

---

Engaging staff in sustainability

Attitudes towards sustainability, and how to address it in a health service, vary. For some healthcare professionals, carbon reduction is an important issue because of concern about their children's future, but others do not believe that climate change is happening. Some staff believe that the health service, or their own part of the health service, is too small to make a difference. However, the experience of the NHS Sustainable Development Unit (SDU) and the Centre for Sustainable Healthcare is that many staff are motivated to change because of the threat of climate change, even those staff who are resistant to appeals to work differently to save money due to the financial plight of the organisation. Suggestions about the ways in which to motivate staff to increase the sustainability of a health service are shown in Box 3.8.

Box 3.8 Ways to motivate staff to increase the sustainability of a health service

- Provide information about the effects of climate change on health
- Describe the factors that contribute to the carbon footprint of a health service
- Ask staff to report what their children are saying about climate change
- Ask how staff are changing their lifestyle to cope with either the threat of climate change or simply the rising cost of energy
- Introduce the concept of 'lean' production, namely, production without waste, because some staff will be motivated by this whatever their views on climate change
- Take part in projects to improve the natural environment of healthcare facilities, for example, the Centre for Sustainable Healthcare runs the NHS Forest, with the aim of planting a tree for every NHS employee

---

Another way of motivating staff is to provide financial and other incentives. Although It may be difficult to identify all the changes resulting from the implementation of a carbon reduction plan because, for example, the electricity used by the ward cannot be identified separately within a hospital's bill, it is usually possible to identify some measures to monitor the decreased use of resources. If carbon savings by a ward or health centre can result in some financial reward, so much the better, but it is also important to appeal to the altruism of staff, encouraging them to take action for the good of society, and the next and future generations including their own children.

Adopting a broad approach to sustainability

It is important to adopt a broad approach to sustainability, considering such aspects as:

- Energy and carbon management;
- Procurement and food;
- Travel, transport and access;
- Water;
- Waste;
- The built environment;
- Organisational and workforce development;
- Partnership and networks;
- Governance;
- Finance.

Imagine you are the director of a maternity service serving a deprived, multi-ethnic population. How would you recruit midwives? One approach is to advertise as widely as your budget allows with the aim of recruiting 'the best', but there are other approaches:

- avoid depleting the midwifery workforces of poor countries as a matter of principle;
- develop a programme in which midwives visit local primary and secondary schools and encourage girls in the surrounding communities to consider midwifery as a career.

Imagine you are a clinical director facing cuts to your budget. One approach is to reduce the costs of support services by outsourcing cleaning and secretarial services. This will reduce your financial costs but at the expense of the income of people who are already the lowest paid in the health service. Another approach is to establish stronger links with the surrounding communities, encouraging the recruitment of local people who are more likely to develop a commitment to the local service and fulfil their responsibilities assiduously irrespective of the level of their salary.

Local sourcing, and not outsourcing, can be applied to other aspects of running a health service. Clinicians could consider promoting the procurement of food from the local foodshed (usually defined as food grown or sourced within a 30-mile radius of the facility). Apart from the environmental benefits of reducing "food miles" and thereby reducing carbon emissions, food sourced locally helps to retain money in the local economy and create wealth in the population served.

The realisation of sustainable development requires long-term planning, which takes into account not only the specific issues relating to healthcare facilities but also factors that could influence the determinants of health. Although addressing the health service's impact on the determinants of health requires a much wider scope than that currently taken by many people who manage healthcare, this type of approach is now recognised as necessary. As *The Lancet* Commission emphasised:

> *Sustainable development also 'includes notions of social justice and equity'.* (22)

Equity is another key responsibility for the clinician practising population medicine, and id discussed in Chapter 4.

Questions for reflection or for use in teaching or network building

If using these questions in network building or teaching, put one of the questions to the group and ask them to work in pairs to reflect on the question for three minutes; try to get people who do not know one another to work together. When taking feedback, let each pair make only one point. In the interests of equity, start with the pair on the left-hand side of the room for responses to the first question, then go to the pair on the right-hand side of the room for responses to the second question.

- What steps can be taken to ensure that increases in productivity actually release cash?
- How can productivity and the need for greater productivity be explained on a local radio programme in 30 seconds?
- Do professionals have a duty to minimise cost?
- How could staff and patient travel be reduced in our service?
- How could we use less energy in heating and lighting in existing buildings, and how can we reduce future energy consumption in any plans for development of the healthcare estate?
- What scope do we have in our services for adopting the four principles of sustainable clinical practice?

References

(1) Ohno, T. (1995) *The Toyota Production System.* Productivity Press
(2) Black, J. and Miller, D. (2008) *The Toyota Way to Healthcare Excellence. Increase Efficiency and Improve Quality with Lean.* ACHE Management Series (p. 236).
(3) Black, J. with Miller, D. (2008) *The Toyota Way to Healthcare Excellence. Increase Efficiency and Improve Quality with Lean.* ACHE Management Series.
(4) Toussaint, J., Gerard, R. And Womack, J. (2010) *On the mend: revolutionizing healthcare to save lives and transform the industry.*
(5) Berwick, D. M. and Hackbarth, A. D. (2012) Eliminating waste in US health care. *Journal of the American Medical Association* 307:1513–1516.
(6) Chief Medical Officer for England (2005) Annual Report.

(7) Nelson, E. C., Batalden, P. B., Godfrey, M. M. (2007) *Quality by Design. A Clinical Microsystems Approach.* John Wiley & Sons Inc. (p. 7).

(8) Sibley, J. C. et al (1982) A randomized trial of continuing medical education *NEJM* 306; 511–515

(9) Chalmers, I. and Glasziou, P. (2009) Avoidable waste in the production and reporting of research evidence. *Lancet* 374: 86–89.

(10) Gallacher, K., Montori V. M. and Mair, F. S. (2011) Understanding Patients' Experiences of Treatment Burden in Chronic Heart Failure Using Normalization Process Theory. *Annals of Family Medicine* 9:235–243.

(11) Department of Health (2009) *Equity and Excellence: Liberating the NHS.*

(12) Claxton, K. et al. (2008) Value-based pricing for NHS drugs: an opportunity not to be missed. *BMJ* 336: 251–5.

(13) Brazier, J., Ratcliffe, J., Salomon, J. A. and Tsuchiya, A. (2007) *Measuring and Valuing Health Benefits for Economic Evaluation.* Oxford University Press.

(14) Mitton, C. and Donaldson, C. (2004) *Priority setting toolkit. A guide to the use of economics in healthcare decision making.* BMJ Publishing Group (p. 47).

(15) Maslach, C. and Leither, M. P. (1997) The truth about burnout. San Francisco: Jossey-Bass. Cited in: Cole, T. R. and Carlin, N. (2009) The art of medicine: the suffering of physicians. *Lancet* 374:1414–15.

(16) Brybye, L. N. and Shanafelt, T. D. (2011) Physician burnout: a Potential Threat to Successful Healthcare Reform. *JAMA* 305;2009–2010

(17) Slim, W. (1956) *Defeat Into Victory.* Cooper Square Press.

(18) NHS Sustainable Development Unit (2009) *Saving Carbon, Improving Health.* NHS Carbon Reduction Strategy for England. January 2009. http://www.sdu.nhs.uk/documents/publications/1237308334_qylG_saving_carbon,_improving_health_nhs_carbon_reducti.pdf

(19) Connor, A. et al. (2010) The carbon footprint of a renal service in the United Kingdom. *Quart. J. Med.* 103: 965–975.

(20) Middleton, J. (2008) Medicine, Conflict and Survival. *Sandwell's Other Health Summit.* 24, Supplement 1: S63

(21) Griffiths, J., Stewart, L. (2008) *Sustaining a healthy future: taking action on climate change.* The Faculty of Public Health, (p. 12).

(22) *Lancet* and University College London Institute for Global Health Commission. (2009) Managing the health effects of climate change. *Lancet* 373: 1693–1733. (p. 1719)

(23) NHS Sustainable Development Unit (2010) *Saving Carbon, Improving Health.* Update. NHS Carbon Reduction Strategy. http://www.sdu.nhs.uk/publications-resources/42/NHS-Carbon-Reduction-Strategy-Update/

(24) Mortimer, F. (2010) The Sustainable Physician. *Clinical Medicine* 10: 110–111.

4

MITIGATING INEQUITY

This chapter will:
- explain the difference between inequity and inequality;
- give examples of ways in which equity can be assessed;
- discuss the relationship of equity in healthcare to the broader issue of social justice.

By the end of the chapter, you will have developed an understanding of:
- how the concepts of equity and social justice are related;
- how to explain the term 'equity' and in what ways it differs from equality;
- how to explore the issue of equity, the Inverse Care Law and unmet need in your service.

Distinguishing inequity from inequality

Many people are confused about the difference between the terms 'inequality' and 'inequity', but the meaning of the two is quite different. Inequality is measured objectively; inequity is a subjective judgement of unfairness.

Health inequalities are measured and reported using criteria such as the standardised mortality ratio (SMR). In all countries, there is marked inequality among different social groups – the greater the level of deprivation the higher the mortality rate. This is clearly depicted in one of the classic visualisations of population health, the Jubilee Line map showing differences in male life-expectancy travelling east from Westminster – every two London Underground stops represent over one year of life-expectancy lost (see Figure 4.1).

The relationship between deprivation and ill-health is well docu-

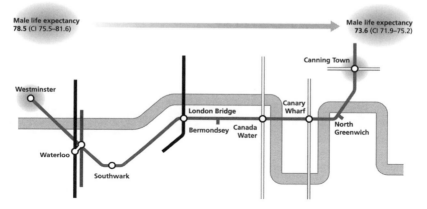

Figure 4.1 Differences in male life-expectancy within a small area of London

mented, and the causal pathway linking the two is mediated through 'the social determinants of health', a term developed and popularised by Michael Marmot (1).

Inequalities in health service provision, however, do not follow the same pattern as inequalities in health. In both the *Dartmouth Atlas of Health Care* and the *NHS Atlases of Variation in Healthcare,*[1] it is obvious that the distribution of many health services bears no consistent relationship to levels of deprivation in populations. There can be marked variation for many aspects of health service provision among similarly wealthy populations and among similarly deprived populations. In the *NHS Atlas of Variation in Healthcare for Children and Young People* (2) and *the NHS Atlas of Variation in Healthcare for Respiratory Disease* (3), several indicators were used to investigate the variation among the 10 most-deprived populations and the 10 least-deprived populations. As can be seen from Figure 4.2, the rate of admissions for bronchiolitis in children per 100,000 population under two years (2008/09–2010/11) shows a 15-fold variation among the 10-most-deprived primary care trusts (PCTs) and a 2.7-fold variation among the 10 least-deprived PCTs.

It is vital that the clinician responsible for population medicine takes account of the health inequalities in the local population. This it

---

[1] http://www.rightcare.nhs.uk/atlas/

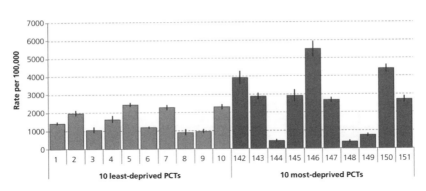

Figure 4.2 Rate of admissions for bronchiolitis in children per 100,000 population under two years: comparison of 10 least-deprived and 10 most-deprived primary care trusts (2008/09–2010/11). (2, 3)

is important because as part of a strategy to improve the health of the whole population it is necessary to try to reduce the level of health inequalities.

> *In fact, recent cross-national evidence suggests that the greater the degree of socio-economic inequality that exists within a society, the steeper the gradient of health inequality. As a result, middle-income groups in a more unequal society will have worse health than comparable or even poorer groups in a society with greater equality. Of course, we cannot infer causation from correlation, but there are plausible hypotheses about pathways which link social inequalities to health, and, even if more work remains to be done to clarify the exact mechanisms, it is not unreasonable to talk here about the social 'determinants' of health.* (4)

As mentioned at the beginning of this chapter, inequality is not the same as inequity. Thomas Rice, a highly respected economist, emphasises the importance of distinguishing between the concepts of equality and equity:

> *The former implies equal shares of something; the latter, a 'fair' or 'just' distribution, which may or may not result in equal shares.* (5)

Classifying inequity in health services

There are several different types of inequity in the provision of health services (see Box 4.1).

Box 4.1 Types of inequity in the provision of health services

- Age-related, when older people are denied treatment simply because of their age
- Gender-related, when women receive effective treatment less frequently than men
- Ethnicity-related, when members of a particular ethnic group receive less care than members of other ethnic groups despite the same level of or greater need as a result of either cultural insensitivity or racism
- Social, when one socio-economic group, almost always the most deprived, does not have the same access to healthcare as other socio-economic groups

---

If there are lower rates of intervention in one subgroup of the population which has the same, or greater, need than the population as a whole, this would suggest there are problems with the equity of provision. If patients in one subgroup of the population receive treatment at a later stage in the course of the disease than patients in another subgroup, this would also suggest problems with the equity of provision. In a study of equity of access to total joint replacement of hip and knee in England, Judge et al. (6) concluded that people in affluent areas got most provision relative to need (see Figure 4.3).

It is also important to be aware that there can be situations in which inequality is equitable. For instance, a health service may decide to provide more resources to a deprived population because the need is greater than that in a less-deprived population.

Process equity should be the goal of health systems. There are several ways in which process equity can be defined.
- *Equal access to health care for equal need*
- *Equal use of health care for equal need*

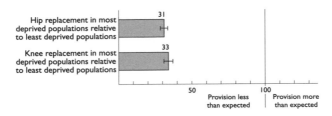

Figure 4.3 Inequities in the provision of hip and knee replacement (6)

- *Equal health care expenditure for equal need.*
All of these refer to equity between people with the same health care needs. This is known as horizontal equity. It is also important to recognize the corollary, that people with different or unequal needs should receive different or unequal health care. This is known as vertical equity. (7)

Another dimension to the concept of healthcare inequity relates to the quality of care provided and not just the volume of care or activity levels. In 1971, Julian Tudor Hart, an exceptional general practitioner, published an article describing the Inverse Care Law, which states that:

the availability of good medical care tends to vary inversely with the need for it in the population served. (8)

A clear illustration of the Inverse Care Law in operation is the experience of single homeless people whose needs are high but who, in most cities, have very poor access to care and therefore receive less high-value care.

Identifying inequity

Some of the root causes of inequity are outwith the power of the medical profession to solve, but the individual clinician with responsibility for a population can mitigate the effects of inequity by identifying people within the population who are likely to be experiencing inequity (see Box 4.2).

Box 4.2 Ways to identify inequity in the population being served

- Compare the number of patients seen from different subgroups within the population, e.g. from different general practices, social groups, or ethnic groups
- Audit referrals to identify differences in levels of need at the point of referral in different groups of patients

---

Having identified inequity, the clinician responsible for a population can take action by:

- making a direct approach to the relevant subgroups in the population, such as engaging with a mosque or church in the locality;
- visiting health centres serving populations from which referrals seem too few.

It is, however, difficult for any clinician to achieve much as an individual. It is important to persuade the healthcare organisation to take action:

- by including representatives of the most deprived subgroups in the population on boards and management groups;
- by investing in the local population, through establishing scholarships at local schools and colleges with the aim of recruiting more local people into the healthcare professions and workforce.

Equity and social justice

It is important for the leadership of any healthcare organisation to appreciate the multidimensional nature of equity; as a concept, it cannot be understood solely in terms of the distribution of healthcare.

Health equity has many aspects, and is best seen as a multidimensional concept. It includes concerns about achievement of health and the capability to achieve good health, not just the distribution of health care. But it also includes the fairness of processes and thus must attach importance to non-discrimina-

tion in the delivery of health care. Furthermore, an adequate engagement with health equity also requires that the considerations of health be integrated with broader issues of social justice and overall equity, paying adequate attention to the versatility of resources and the diverse reach and impact of different social arrangements.' (9)

Equity is a matter of social justice, and any publicly funded health service has a part to play in creating a just society as well as a healthy society; indeed, some would argue that a population cannot be healthy if there is significant injustice.

Justice . . . requires meeting health care needs fairly under resource constraints and this, in turn, requires limiting care in a publicly accountable way. (10)

Taking this perspective, health promotion encompasses efforts not only to change individuals' lifestyles but also to promote social justice.

Questions for reflection or for use in teaching or network building

If using these questions in network building or teaching, put one of the questions to the group and ask them to work in pairs to reflect on the question for three minutes; try to get people who do not know one another to work together. When taking feedback, let each pair make only one point. In the interests of equity, start with the pair on the left-hand side of the room for responses to the first question, then go to the pair on the right-hand side of the room for responses to the second question.

- What can be done by the NHS to tackle inequity in access to healthcare when the causes of inequity are so deeply embedded in society?
- When considering your service, which subgroups in the local population are at greatest risk of inequity?
- What could you do next year to reduce inequity in your service?

References

(1) WHO (2008) Closing the gap in a generation: Health equity through action on the social determinants of health; report of the Commission chaired by Michael Marmot

(2) Right Care (2012) NHS Atlas of Variation in Healthcare for Children and Young People. Reducing unwarranted variation to increase value and improve quality. March 2012. http://www.rightcare.nhs.uk/atlas/

(3) Right Care (2012) NHS Atlas of Variation in Healthcare for People with Respiratory Disease. Reducing unwarranted variation to increase value and improve quality. September 2012. http://www.rightcare.nhs.uk/atlas/

(4) Daniels, N., Kennedy, B. and Kawachi, I. (2004) Health and Inequality, or, Why Justice is Good for Our Health. In: Anand, S., Peter, F. and Sen, A. *Public Health, Ethics, and Equity.* Oxford University Press (p. 63).

(5) Rice, T. (1998) *The Economics of Health Reconsidered.* Health Administration Press (p. 152).

(6) Judge, A. et al. (2010) Equity in access to total joint replacement of hip and knee in England. *Br. Med. J.* doi 10/1136bmj.c4902.

(7) Wonderling, D., Gruen, R. and Black, N. (2005) *Introduction to Health Economics. Understanding Public Health.* Open University Press (p. 157).

(8) Hart, J. T. (1971) The Inverse Care Law. *Lancet* 392: 48–49.

(9) Sen, A. (2004) Why Health Equity? In: Anand, S., Peter, F. and Sen, A. (Eds) *Public Health, Ethics, and Equity.* Oxford University Press (p. 31).

(10) Daniels, N. and Sabin, J. (2008) Setting Limits Fairly. Learning to share resources for health. Second edition. Oxford University Press (p. 13).

5

PROMOTING HEALTH AND PREVENTING DISEASE

This chapter will:
- offer several definitions of health;
- describe the relationship between health equity and justice;
- explain the part that a clinician can play in disease prevention.

By the end of the chapter, you will have developed an understanding of:
- why every health service must play a part in disease prevention;
- how hospital health services can contribute to improving health;
- whether the clinician practising population medicine has a responsibility for advocacy on behalf of the population's health

The meanings of 'health'

The meaning of the term 'health' is problematic and under continuous evolution. However, there is a general consensus that a health service in isolation cannot promote health and prevent disease because it has no operational jurisdiction over almost all of the social determinants of health. Although all clinicians have a responsibility to promote health and prevent disease by providing information and support to the individual patients who consult them, this responsibility is of equal or greater significance for the clinician practising population medicine.

The well-known definition of health enshrined in the WHO Constitution of 1948 serves a useful function:

Health is a complete state of physical, mental and social well-being and not merely the absence of disease or infirmity. (1)

Some authorities, however, argue that this definition is too narrow. For Amartya Sen, the concept of health should encompass two other concepts:

- social justice;
- the societal responsibility to ensure that every individual has the capability of achieving their full potential (2).

Other distinguished philosophers, notably Norman Daniels, argue that this type of very broad definition is not useful.

> *I shall follow Boorse's (1997) suggestion and say that health is the absence of pathology. (Admittedly, 'health is the absence of pathology' has neither the ring nor the familiarity of 'health is the absence of disease'.) We may understand 'pathology' to refer to any deviation from the natural functional organization of a typical member of a species . . . is a departure from normal functioning . . . Before saying more about understanding health as normal function, I want to forestall a common misunderstanding about the narrowness of this biomedical conception. The conceptual narrowness is required. Health is not all there is to well-being or happiness, contrary to the famous World Health Organization (WHO) definition: 'Health is a state of complete physical, mental, and social well-being, and not merely the absence of disease or infirmity.' The WHO definition risks turning all of social philosophy and social policy into health care. (3)*

If we focus on Daniels' definition of health, which is narrower than that of Sen, it becomes all the more apparent that health services whose primary function is the diagnosis and treatment of disease should be involved in promoting and protecting the health of the population they serve, especially when the definitions given below are used to guide health service activity.

> *Health promotion comprises efforts to enhance positive health and reduce the risk of ill-health. (4)*

> *Health protection comprises legal or fiscal controls, other regulations and policies, and voluntary codes of practice. (4)*

From Sen's perspective, health workers should be concerned about social injustice even if it does not cause disease or complicate treatment, whereas Daniels' definition means that health workers should focus on injustice and inequity only when they are complicating factors in the prevention or treatment of disease.

The clinician's contribution

In some countries, public health professionals view public health as a medical specialty. In other countries, in addition to the organisation of primary and secondary preventive services (e.g. smoking cessation and screening, respectively), public health professionals focus on environmental protection or interpret their role as one of advocacy for social change.

However, clinicians primarily involved in diagnosis, treatment and care can also have a very important role to play in disease prevention. Although the public health professional is trained in the effective delivery of preventive services, the clinician has charismatic authority. While a public health professional may have charismatic authority, it tends to carry less impact with the general public and partner organisations. For instance, a report by a well-respected public health professional will have less effect than a media interview with a doctor in a white coat or scrubs. The impact of a trainee surgeon speaking about knife wounds, an emergency room specialist testifying to the terrible consequences of binge drinking, and a lung specialist holding a cancerous lung in a bottle needs to be harnessed more often.

However, there are many less dramatic steps that can be taken by a clinician practising population medicine in order to prevent disease, for example, by ensuring that:

- everyone with heart disease, and not just those referred, are receiving aspirin and other evidence-based measures to control risk factors for a recurrent heart attack;
- every person with chronic lung and heart disease is receiving flu immunisation;
- every individual with tuberculosis is supported during the course of therapy until they have been cured;

- all the relatives of people diagnosed with familial hyper-cholesterolaemia are identified and invited for testing.

Preventive healthcare is the most sustainable type of healthcare, but it requires focus and coordination, not only by public health professionals but also by practitioners of population medicine. Although some hospitals are now appointing public health professionals, this does not reduce the need for clinicians to be responsible for, and take action to improve, the health of the whole population.

Authority, leadership and action

Clinicians with management responsibilities have bureaucratic authority within the institution at which they fulfil those responsibilities. Clinicians practising population medicine will have some bureaucratic authority, but to fulfil their responsibilities they will have to employ other forms of authority:

- sapiential authority, derived from their knowledge;
- charismatic authority, derived from their leadership position.

> *Management is a set of processes that can keep a complicated system of people and technology running smoothly. The most important aspects of management include planning, budgeting, organizing, staffing, controlling, and problem solving. Leadership is a set of processes that creates organizations in the first place or adapts them to significantly changing circumstances. Leadership defines what the future should look like, aligns people with that vision, and inspires them to make it happen despite the obstacles. (5)*

Management is mainly a transactional process, whereas leadership should be transformational, and not simply transactional. Thus, a leader not only has to deliver results but also has to transform organisations that serve the population. Transformational leadership may require that a clinician responsible for population medicine tries to improve the prevention of disease through advocacy:

- by visiting the local Member of Parliament (MP);

- by seeking to influence directly national or international policy-making;
- by ensuring that the relevant professional organisation is fully engaged in debates and decisions that could reduce the risk of disease.

As the line of accountability in population medicine is to the population served and not to the Chief Executive of a bureaucracy, the clinician practising population medicine may need to take action without seeking permission and should remember the old adage 'It is easier to seek forgiveness than permission'. For instance, it would be appropriate for a clinician to brief a local Member of Parliament on the need for alcohol legislation without first asking the Chief Executive's permission, but it would be inappropriate to criticise the organisation to which they belong unless they had attempted to achieve change in the first place before deciding to 'blow the whsitle'.

Hospitals as health services

Language creates the culture within which people make decisions and express various behaviours. The traditional bureaucratic division of health services and the language used to describe these services – 'hospital' and 'community' in relation to care and the separate identification of 'mental health services' – creates the wrong culture, one in which the hospital is assumed to be outside the community and only in the healthcare and not the health business (see Figure 5.1). Hospital services, however, can play a major role in improving health the health of the populations they serve, and acting as a public health service.

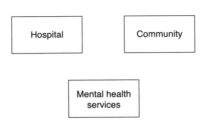

Figure 5.1 Healthcare as an archipelago

'Public health' is another term that causes confusion because it is, in one sense, a description of a professional group, in another the outcome of the efforts of everyone seeking to prevent, diagnose and treat disease and promote health. Some hospitals are now setting up public health departments which have public health professionals within them, an approach sometimes called 'the health-promoting hospital'. These departments sometimes focus on ensuring that every person who comes into hospital as a patient receives help to stop smoking. Although such moves are welcome, it is important not to create the impression that it absolves every other department in the hospital from using their opportunities and influence to promote health and prevent disease. Every hospital department has the ability to influence the health of the population served:

- the trauma team can campaign against knife crime;
- the hepatology service can campaign against harmful and hazardous drinking;
- the cardiology service can promote exercise and physical activity.

In addition, the hospital as a whole can contribute to improving the health of the population it serves. For instance, in South Auckland, the Middlemore Hospital decided not to recruit more nurses and health workers from the Philippines or Thailand but instead set up a Health Academy to inspire young people from the Maori and Pasifika communities to aspire to become health workers at Middlemore with great success.

Questions for reflection or for use in teaching or network building

If using these questions in network building or teaching, put one of the questions to the group and ask them to work in pairs to reflect on the question for three minutes; try to get people who do not know one another to work together. When taking feedback, let each pair make only one point. In the interests of equity, start with the pair on the left-hand side of the room for responses to the first question, then go to the pair on the right-hand side of the room for responses to the second question.

- What is the most useful definition of health for a clinical service?
- How could a musculo-skeletal or mental health service contribute to the prevention of disease?
- What are the advocacy responsibilities of clinician practising population medicine?
- In what ways could a clinician ensure that locally and nationally elected representatives are adequately informed on population health issues?

References

(1) World Health Organization (WHO) Preamble to the Constitution of the World Health Organization as adopted by the International Health Conference, New York, 19 June–22 July 1946; signed on 22 July 1946 by the representatives of 61 States (Official Records of the World Health Organization, no. 2, p. 100) and entered into force on 7 April 1948. http://www.who.int/suggestions/faq/en/index.html
(2) Sen, A. (2004) Why Health Equity? In: Anand, S., Peter, F. and Sen, A. (Eds) *Public Health, Ethics, and Equity.* Oxford University Press.
(3) Daniels, N. (2008) Just Health. *Meeting health needs fairly.* Cambridge University Press.
(4) Downie, R. S., Tannahill, C. and Tannahill, A. (1996) *Health Promotion. Models and Values.* Second edition. Oxford University Press.
(5) Kotter, J. (1996) *Leading Change.* Harvard Business School Press.

6

DESIGNING POPULATION-BASED INTEGRATED SYSTEMS

This chapter will:

- explain the difference between a system and an institution;
- define the basic components of a system, including the aim and objectives;
- describe each component of a system using examples as relevant;
- distinguish between individual outcomes and population outcomes.

By the end of this chapter, you will have developed an understanding of:

- the way in which the objectives for a system differ from the aim of a system;
- the way in which objectives can be set;
- the different types of criteria or measures that can be used to assess progress towards meeting the objectives;
- the way in which standards for a system can be set.
- The 20th century was the century of the institution; the 21st century is the century of the system.

From great institutions to great systems

In the Middle Ages, people built cathedrals; in the 19th century, they built railway stations; in the 20th century, they built hospitals. These hospitals became the great institutions of the 20th century, and the powerful and wealthy became members of hospital boards, similar to the way in which they had supported the Church in an earlier era, although few hospitals can hold a candle to the architectural glories of Notre Dame in Paris or St Pancras Station in London. Many hospitals are huge, sprawling sites, continually evolving and never reaching completion, like Sagrada Familia.

Hospitals became the sites for the delivery of specialist services, and also sites for the development of super-specialist services; these services came to be called secondary and tertiary care, respectively. In addition, mental health services developed in the 19th century, most obviously in the form of asylums located on the edge of towns and cities remote from the hospitals, even though many of the residents had physical as well as mental problems, as is the case today.

In the second half of the 20th century, two new institutions developed – general practice and government-run community services. General practice evolved from being composed of isolated practitioners in private practice to becoming a powerful force with the establishment of a Royal College and the development of an evidence base, in part as a consequence of the funding provided by the NHS. Community services provided voluntary and charitable services that had cared for the elderly, the infirm and children.

The situation now, not only in the United Kingdom, is that healthcare is an archipelago with four great islands connected by the occasional ferry (Figure 6.1).

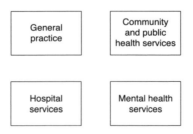

Figure 6.1 The healthcare archipelago

By the end of the 20th century there was also growing concern about the need to develop an integrated approach to common health problems through defining systems of care (1). The exemplar of an integrated system of care is that for people with cancer. Faced with the considerable capital expense of providing radiotherapy, the managers of most district general hospitals accepted that investment in that intervention should take place in teaching hospitals. This intensity of investment at some but not all healthcare site led to the creation of cancer networks, across which were delivered a system of care ranging from screening to end-of-life care. Constraints on capital investment also led to the development of systems for:

- end-stage renal failure;
- acute stroke;
- myocardial infarction.

In a population-based system, the archipelago of care is transformed into a set of inter-related types of care which recognises that self-care is the most important (Figure 6.2).

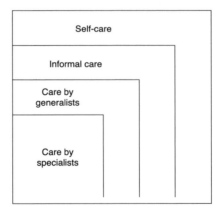

Figure 6.2 Four-box healthcare

Each system of care needs to have a focus. The various types of system focus for health services in countries with developed economies are shown in Box 6.1.

There can be tension between generalists and specialists but it is possible to minimise any tension by being clear about the relationship between complex and complicated health problems.

When discussing a condition such as asthma or epilepsy, it is common for general practitioners to point out that many of their

---

Box 6.1 The various types of focus for systems of care

- Symptoms or clinical presentations, such as breathlessness or back pain
- Diseases or conditions, such as inflammatory bowel disease, asthma or depression
- Subgroups of the population, such as frail elderly people or people under the 65 years of age with multiple morbidities

---

patients have more than one problem. Indeed, people with multiple morbidities, often physical, mental and social, have complex problems – for example, an 84-year-old woman with four diagnoses and seven prescriptions being supported by a 50-year-old daughter with depression and a husband with an alcohol abuse problem. This is a complex problem but it is common in general practice. However, when one of the older woman's four problems, heart failure, for example, becomes complicated, the generalist needs to seek specialist advice. This highlights the relationship between complex and complicated problems, between the roles of generalist and specialist.

By contrast, in low- and middle-income countries, there is a move to create integrated primary care due to the inefficiencies that result from a collection of disease-based systems, such as onchocerciasis or malaria, which operate in isolation.

The development of systems of care does not reduce the need for good management of healthcare institutions, but it does require the skill to create and manage what have been called hybrid organisations, defined as organisations in which:

> . . . functional units and mission orientated units work together and the accompanying principle of dual reporting, like a democracy, are not great in and of themselves. They just happen to be the best way for any business to be organised. (2)

Other people call this arrangement 'matrix management' and the pattern is emerging in many countries (see Matrix 6.1).

Andy Grove, who developed the definition of a hybrid organisation, was the Chief Executive of Intel and could control both dimensions of

Matrix 6.1

		SYSTEMS					
		Cancer	Respiratory	Mental Health	Stroke	Frail Elderly	Children
FACILITIES	HR						
	Transport						
	Finance						
	Real Estate						
	IT						

the matrix. The situation is more complex in healthcare where the contributions of different autonomous organisations must be integrated. This challenge requires the development of networks which will be discussed in Chapter 7.

The definition and design of a system

A system is a set of activities with a common set of objectives. To expand this definition, a system is a set of activities with a common aim and set of objectives, which produces an annual report for the population served, using criteria and standards common to all systems with the same focus.

The design and development of systems of care is described in detail in the companion book *How to Build Healthcare Systems*. The principal points in that book have been summarised in this chapter but some different examples have been used so the reader of this text will find new material. The design of a system has several stages (see Box 6.2). For the rest of this chapter, the first five stages in the process of designing and developing a system will be described, including the practical steps that can be taken at each stage. To accomplish the first five stages in the process, it will require several meetings of the team responsible for system development, at least five meetings of various stakeholders who will be involved in delivering the system of care under development, and time for wider consultation between stakeholder meetings.

The team responsible for system development should have representation from all the key organisations, and consultation should include other people who will be important in making sure the design is implemented. All the organisations and people involved in implementation comprise the network.

Box 6.2 Stages in the design of a system of care

- Define the scope of the system
- Define the population for which the system has responsibility
- Reach agreement on the aim and objectives for the system
- For each objective, select one or more criteria with which to measure progress
- For each objective, set standards to enable benchmarking and comparison among services
- Reach agreement on the network of organisations necessary to deliver and govern the system (see Chapter 7)
- Identify the resources necessary to create a budget for the system (see Chapter 9)

Defining the scope of the system

It is important to be aware that people may express in an unfocussed way and terms such as 'frail elderly' are used frequently without ever being clarified and agreed.

To define the scope of a system, it is essential to identify the set of activities that need to be coordinated through the system. The scope should be as wide as is necessary to include every activity relevant to the aim. The team leading the development of the system are responsible for facilitating agreement on the activities to be included in the scope. Part of this facilitation process could involve testing or clarifying the boundaries of the scope through posing a series of questions (see Table 6.1).

Table 6.1 Questions to clarify the scope of a system in relation to the system focus

System focus	Questions to clarify scope boundaries
Frail elderly people	• Should we use an arbitrary indicator such as being on four medications? • Should we simply include everyone in a nursing home? • Should we use a predictive risk score? • Should we include everyone with dementia? • Does it include end-of-life care?
Children	• Should we include neonates or should they be included in the scope for the maternity system? • What is the upper age limit for children to be covered by the system? • Is it better to establish a linked system for young people in transition, perhaps for those aged 15–24 years?
Musculo-skeletal programme	• Are people with fractures included in this system? • Should there be a separate sub-system for people requiring joint replacement?

It is usually better to start with a subgroup of the population such as 'people at the end of life', rather than a service such as 'palliative care'. Using this approach, the real issue can be identified. For example, a discussion intended to develop an urgent care system quickly evolved into a focus on people with multiple morbidities, including both elderly (the 'frail elderly'), and people under 65 years who have considerable mental health and substance abuse problems. Sometimes a Venn diagram is more useful than a list (Figure 6.3).

Having defined the scope of the system, the next step is to define the population to be served.

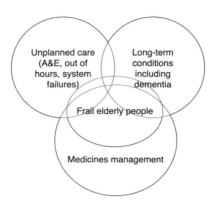

Figure 6.3 The subgroups that make up the 'frail elderly' population

Defining the population to be served

Each system of care has responsibility for a defined population. However, it is not always clear what should constitute the defined population for a particular system. For instance, although a population may appear to be clearly defined by a political jurisdiction such as a local authority, it is essential to define the population boundaries for a system of care because clinical communities of practice do not often correspond to politically defined jurisdictions. One way to define the population served by a system of care in the NHS is to 'construct' it from the relevant general practice populations given that general practices are responsible for the small populations that constitute the larger population. In countries in which insurance schemes ensure population coverage, the members of the scheme becomes the population.

At this stage, it is important to decide upon the optimum size of the population to be served by the system. In the traditional model of institution-based care, the size of the population served is about 300,000 people, based on the catchment population for a general hospital. The optimum population size for a system of care, however, is a function of several inter-related variables:

1. the incidence and prevalence of the problem – the size of the population must be large enough to include the number of clinical

events sufficient to enable clinical expertise to be developed and for the production of a meaningful annual report;

2. the level of population need for super-specialist services and technology, such as neurosurgery.

The implications of two of these variables for optimum population size in relation to several different systems of care are shown in Table 6.2.

Table 6.2 The optimum size of population for a system

System focus	Incidence and prevalence	Population need for super-specialist intervention	Optimum population size
Asthma	High	Low	200,000–500,000
Epilepsy	High	High	There may need to be both a local support service for a smaller population – 300,000 – and a neurosurgical service related to a larger population – 1 or 2 million – so that the local service's referral rates can be compared
Parkinson's disease	High	Low	300,000–500,000, although the need for deep brain stimulation may require a larger population size
Frail elderly people	High	Low	200,000–500,000
Motor neurone disease	Low	High	Support for this uncommon condition requires specialist teams

Reaching agreement on the aim and objectives

Aim: A high-level statement of the role of the department. (3)

Every system of care should have a single high-level aim with which all professionals and patients can identify. Examples of high-level aims are shown in Display 6.1.

Display 6.1 Examples of aims

Organisation	Aim
NASA	To put a man on the moon and bring him safely back (12 words)
National Breast Cancer Screening Programme	To offer women the opportunity of reducing their risk of dying from breast cancer (14 words)
A hospital	To offer high-quality, safe care tailored to meet the needs of each individual (13 words)

However, the aim of a system has to be complemented by a set of more detailed objectives on which everyone involved in providing care can focus their activities.

Objectives are needed in every area where performance and results directly and vitally affect the survival and prosperity of the business. . . . Objectives should enable us to do five things:

- *to organize and explain the whole range of business phenomena in a small number of general statements;*
- *to test these statements in actual experience;*
- *to predict behaviour;*
- *to appraise the soundness of decisions when they are still being made; and*
- *to enable practising businessmen to analyse their own experience and, as a result, improve their performance.*

A draft set of objectives for a system for liver disease developed in a workshop is set out in Box 6.3.

Box 6.3 Draft set of objectives for a Liver Disease Programme

- To diagnose and treat liver disease quickly and accurately
- To treat liver disease effectively and safely
- To engage people with the condition and their carers as equal partners
- To promote the health of people with liver disease
- To develop the professionals who support people with liver disease
- To make the best use of resources
- To promote and support research
- To produce an annual report for the population served

There are two main types of objectives for a system of care:

1. 'clinical' objectives, which are analogues of traditional clinical activity, such as to diagnose accurately and quickly;
2. population objectives, relating to the use of resources for the whole population; population objectives are often overlooked by clinicians when setting the objectives for a system.

Practical steps involved in the development of a high-level aim for a system of care are shown in Box 6.4, and the practical steps involved in reaching agreement on the objectives for that system are shown in Box 6.5. At the same meeting, the group responsible for system development should also draft and agree a set of objectives.

During the process of objective-setting, the scope may need to be changed. For example, when the draft set of objectives for liver disease were discussed in a workshop run by public health professionals, an objective to prevent liver disease, was introduced as follows:

To prevent alcoholic liver disease, principally by changing culture and the environment

---

Box 6.4 Practical steps in the development of an aim for a system

- Hold a meeting of the management team
- Give the team the examples of aims shown in Box 6.3
- Ask people to work in pairs for 3 minutes to draft an aim for the system in development; then ask each pair for suggestions during feedback – it may be possible to reach agreement on a draft aim after one round of feedback but two or more rounds may be needed
- After feedback, draft an aim – redraft it if necessary and reach agreement; try to keep the length to under 25 words
- Circulate the draft aim to a wide range of stakeholders who will be involved in the system; give stakeholders and participants who attended the drafting meeting a month in which to respond
- Redraft the aim in the light of responses and suggested amendments

---

Box 6.5 Practical steps in the development of a set of objectives for a system

- Remind the group of the system aim that was previously agreed
- Consider circulating a draft set of objectives for another condition, for example, the objectives shown in Box 6.3 could be used, but from experience it is better to let people think freely
- Ask people to work in pairs to identify at least one objective for the system in development
- Take feedback
- Type up the responses during a refreshment break
- At this stage, it may be necessary to introduce population-type objectives

Present the set of objectives and facilitate a discussion on each to reach an agreement on wording

---

Choosing criteria

For each objective, there should be one or more criteria associated with it to enable progress towards the objective to be measured.

Choosing criteria is a more time-consuming process and may need to be addressed separately. For instance, it is important to reach an agreed definition of what is meant by certain phrases 'to diagnose quickly' and 'to diagnose accurately'.

Each objective needs to have one or more criteria associated with it in order to measure progress. Without criteria, objectives are meaningless.

Several terms are used as synonyms for 'criteria', such as 'metrics', 'indicators', or 'measures'. Some people use the term 'measures' to mean criteria that are considered to be of greater validity than indicators; for example, they would use the term 'measure' about systematic surveys of patient experience, whereas they would use the word 'indicator' for the number of letters of complaint or commendation that a hospital Chief Executive received. Although the latter is less costly, it is less valuable in terms of feedback for the system than the accurate measures used in the former.

Similar issues tend to be raised in any discussion about criteria that could be used to measure progress, including:

- The availability of data;
- The validity of criteria;
- Whether to use process or outcome criteria.

Availability of data

The data already being collected are rarely those needed to provide the information required to monitor progress, because originally they were selected for another specific reason. When selecting criteria, it is important not to be constrained by data availability, but to determine the criterion required to monitor each objective and then to specify the data needed to enable the measure to be calculated. For instance, if the criterion is related to the objective of diagnosing rheumatoid arthritis quickly, the data needed are:

- the date of first presentation with joint pain;

- the date of definitive diagnosis.

These data may be from different databases, the former in general practice records, of which there may be many of different types, the latter in hospital pharmacy records. In the past, this would have been a major problem because a new 'information system' would have had to be commissioned. Nowadays, and in future, however, the power of cloud computing, namely the ability to use the Internet as the storage system, enables data to be extracted from different sources.

Validity of criteria

The validity of a criterion is the degree to which it actually measures the change it purports to measure. For example, if one objective is to provide a service that patients value, the number of complaints received is of lower validity than a survey of all patients, although the latter is more time-consuming and more expensive to undertake. This example demonstrates the trade-off between validity and feasibility: for a criterion with a high level of validity, the data are usually more difficult to collect than those for a criterion with a relatively low level of validity. If, however, the data for a criterion with a high level of validity become part of routine data collection, then services can be monitored using appropriate and what would usually be viewed as sophisticated measures. For instance, at the Dartmouth Hitchcock Medical Center, the preferences of each woman considering breast cancer treatment options are routinely collected which means that their recorded preference can then be compared with the treatment they actually receive.

Process or outcome criteria?

For decades, the provision of health services was measured using classic economic criteria such as the amount of resource invested or the volume of work done, i.e. inputs and outputs. In the 1960s, however, Avedis Donabedian published his work on quality assurance (5), and introduced a different nomenclature from that of the economists (see Table 6.3).

Table 6.3 A comparison of classic economic terminology and Donabedian's terminology in relation to healthcare criteria

Criterion	Economic terminology	Donabedian's terminology
Number of beds in surgical wards	Inputs	Structure
Number of operations in a year	Outputs	Process
Percentage of patients whose operation was a success	Not considered originally	Outcome
Use of resources	Outputs/inputs = productivity	Outcomes/inputs = efficiency

In the years following Donabedian's publication, there has been much discussion about the relative merits of process and outcome measures. Some authorities are proponents of outcome measures, whereas others support the use of process measures for the reason given by Porter.

There is a particular problem with outcomes in that it is often difficult to attribute a given outcome improvement (such as in the health of a patient) to a particular item of public service (such as a course of medical treatment), for the outcome may in large part be due to a variety of factors that are not within the control of the providers of the service concerned (such as the patient's own recuperative powers). This is one of the reasons why, although both providers and policy-makers often pay lip service to the important of outcomes, in practice they usually give more attention to factors that are more under the control of the service, such as inputs, processes and outputs. (6)

Currently, the trend is towards the measurement of outcomes, even if the criteria most readily available and easiest to collect are process measures.

Health outcomes refer to objective results, not just physician or patient perceptions of outcomes. There is not just one outcome of the care for any health condition, but multiple outcomes that jointly constitute value. Patient circumstances and preferences will affect the weighting of these outcomes to some degree.... (7)

However, it is necessary to collect both outcome and process measures. Process measures remain important for two reasons:

1. the outcome of a service may not become apparent for years, rendering it unsuitable as a criterion for day-to-day management. The outcome of a breast cancer screening programme – such as a decline in mortality – will not become evident, even at a national level, for years, whereas the person responsible for managing a screening programme needs to know the outcome on an annual, monthly and sometimes, in the case of radiation levels, daily basis;
2. the outcome may be determined by factors other than the quality of the service.

The practical steps that can be undertaken to select criteria for the monitoring of system objectives are shown in Box 6.6.

Setting standards

A standard: the level of compliance with a criterion or indicator, for example 90% of patients in a practice with a blood pressure of more than 160/90 should have their blood pressure remeasured within three months. (8)

It is possible to set standards for a single system of care using the criteria and outcomes that have been agreed, including:

- an excellent standard, the performance of the best service;
- a minimal acceptable standard, below which the system does not wish to fall;
- an achievable standard which can be arbitrarily, but usefully, set by choosing the cut-off point between the top quintile and the bottom three quintiles (Figure 6.4)

However, it is much better if several systems of care or services work together to set standards. One of the objectives of standard-setting is to help services improve their quality of care by competing with other

---

Box 6.6 Practical steps in the selection of criteria to monitor objectives in a system of care

- Invite the group involved in system development, involved in setting the objectives, and people with experience in designing research projects even if they are not doing research on the topic, their expertise in the definition and measurement of outcomes will be very helpful
- Prior to the meeting, conduct a structured literature search to identify outcome measures that are already available for the system focus
- If outcome measures are already available, in the meeting, consider whether to supplement them with outcomes of importance to your community of practice
- At the meeting, for each objective, ask participants to suggest the process criterion or criteria they would use to measure progress; remind them not to take account at this stage of the availability or difficulty of obtaining the data necessary for monitoring
- Ask the professionals what constitutes a good outcome from their perspective and record the responses
- Ask the patients what constitutes a good outcome from their perspective and record the responses
- Ask the professionals what constitutes a bad outcome from their perspective and record the responses
- Ask the patients what constitutes a bad outcome from their perspective and record the responses
- Ask the researchers to comment and advise on the responses of both professionals and patients
- Collate the responses about criteria, try to reach a consensus and record the conclusions
- Identify the data items associated with each criterion that are required to measure progress against the objectives, and specify the details relating to the data needed, the data collection cycle, and the adaptations to routine data systems that are necessary to enable data collection

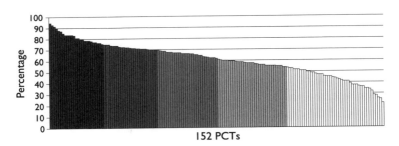

Figure 6.4 Percentage of patients admitted to hospital following a stroke who spend 90% of their time on a stroke unit by primary care trust (PCT) in England (2009/10)(9)

services, using the standards as the benchmark. Standard-setting requires several services to apply the same objectives, criteria and standards – namely, to have a common system of care. If nationally agreed standards are available, these should be used; if there are no nationally agreed standards, follow the steps shown in Box 6.7.

Once the system has been designed, the next stage is to build it. Building a system requires the development of a network of key organisations responsible for delivering care to the population.

Box 6.7 Practical steps towards standard-setting for a system of care

- Convene a meeting of the clinicians responsible for the population-based systems of care
- Prior to the meeting, identify the system objectives for which there are pre-existing good-quality performance information because, if possible, standards should be set using data that reflect the current situation across all the services; circulate this information prior to the meeting, but also ensure it is available at the meeting
- At the meeting, ask participants to consider the performance data for all the services, and to identify the performance level that constitutes a minimal acceptable standard for each objective
- Returning to the performance data, ask participants to identify the performance level that distinguishes the top quartile of services from the rest; agree this as the achievable standard towards which all services in the other three quartiles should aspire, the services in the top quartile to aspire to match, and the best performing service to try to do even better
- If there are no data that can be compared, ask participants to develop minimal acceptable and achievable standards based on their knowledge and experience

---

Questions for reflection or for use in teaching or network building

If using these questions in network building or teaching, put one of the questions to the group and ask them to work in pairs to reflect on the question for three minutes; try to get people who do not know one another to work together. When taking feedback, let each pair make only one point. In the interests of equity, start with the pair on the left-hand side of the room for responses to the first question, then go to the pair on the right-hand side of the room for responses to the second question.

- What are the main obstacles to the introduction and development of systems in healthcare?
- Identify five services including one that is diagnostic in which you are involved or which you know about, e.g. a service for women with pelvic pain. Give each of these services a score on a scale from 1 to 10, where 1 is chaos and 10 represents a perfect system.
- List three things that institutions are good at doing in healthcare and three things that they fail to do

---

References

(1) Gray, J. A. M. (1983) Four Box Healthcare: Planning in a Time of Zero Growth. *Lancet* 2: 1185–6.

(2) Grove, A. S. (1995) *High output management.* Vintage Books. (p136.)

(3) Scrivens, E. (2005) *Quality, Risk and Control in Health Care.* Open University Press (p. 91).

(4) Drucker, P. (1955) *The Practice of Management.* Elsevier, Butterworth-Heinemann (pp. 54–5).

(5) Donabedian, A. (2003) *Introduction to Quality Assurance in Healthcare.* Oxford.

(6) Porter, M. E. (2008) What is Value in Health Care? Harvard Business School. Institute for Strategy and competitiveness. White Paper

(7) Neumann, P. J., Tunis, S. R. (2010) Medicare and Medical Technology – the Growing Demand for Relevant Outcomes. *New Eng. J. Med.* 362: 5: 377.

(8) Grol, M., Baker, R., Moss, F. (2004) *Quality Improvement Research.* BMJ Books.

(9) Right Care (2010) NHS Atlas of Variation in Healthcare. Reducing unwarranted variation to increase value and improve quality. November 2010 (p. 48). http://www.rightcare.nhs.uk/atlas/

7

CREATING NETWORKS TO DELIVER SYSTEMS

This chapter will:

- define networks and networking;
- describe the principles of network management;
- summarise steps that can be taken to build sustainable networks;
- give examples of different types of networks, classified by the degree of managerial formality;
- describe interventions that can be used to develop or strengthen the network;
- describe the need for explicit pathways that patients can follow through the network.

By the end of this chapter, you will have developed an understanding of:

- the difference between a network and a hierarchy;
- the relative contributions of institutions and systems;
- how to build a network;
- how to sustain and develop a network;
- the contribution that networks make to delivering systems of care;
- the role of a network coordinator;
- the difference between a network and a team;
- the contribution that pathways make to standardise and personalise care.

Once a system of care has been designed, the next step is to deliver it to the population in need. There are two principal ways in which change is brought about within a health service – through people or through the organisation, each of which comprises three elements (see Figure 7.1).

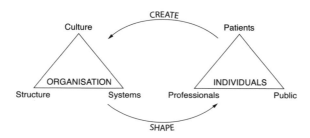

Figure 7.1 The two elements of a health service – the people and the organisation

For the last 50 years, those who pay for or manage health services have sought to achieve change principally by changing the structure of the organisation, given that it can take years or decades for education to have an effect.

The need to shift the focus from structure

Organizing is the process of arranging collective effort so that it achieves an outcome potentially superior to that of individuals acting or working alone. It almost always involves some division of labor, with different people or groups concentrating on different activities that have to be integrated (co-ordinated) to achieve a successful result. (1)

In seeking to change the organisation of healthcare, priority has previously been given to changing the structure:

- by re-organising the bureaucracy;
- by introducing a market;
- by both re-organisation and the introduction of a market.

In this book, it is argued that priority should be given to the development of population-based and integrated systems of care rather than to structural change. Indeed, there is a growing consensus that a new form of organisation is needed to deliver a system of care.

This new form is known as a network, and will become the dominant type of organisation in the 21st century, displacing, but not rendering redundant, the bureaucracy, the dominant type of organisation in the 20th century.

As health services grew in size during the 20th century, it became clear that clinicians needed an organisation to support them. The type of organisation that flourished in every country's health service was the bureaucracy, much criticised by those who have experienced only bad bureaucracy. Bureaucratisation, however, can bring several benefits.

> *'Bureaucracy' is a dirty word, both to the average person and to many specialists on organizations. It suggests rigid rules and regulations, a hierarchy of offices, narrow specialization of personnel, an abundance of offices or units which can hamstring those who want to get things done, impersonality, resistance to change. Yet every organization of any significant size is bureaucratized to some degree or, to put it differently, exhibits more or less stable patterns of behaviour based upon a structure of roles and specialized tasks. Bureaucracy, in this sense, is another word for structure. (2)*

Although bureaucracies are necessary, they can develop in ways that are unhelpful if they have misguided leadership. One manifestation of over-bureaucratisation is an emphasis on hierarchy, i.e. 'a system of nested groups' (3), in which senior managers operate in what is known as 'command and control' mode.

Markets have also been introduced to varying degrees in the organisation of health services in many countries: in the United States, the role of the market is extensive, whereas in Canada that role is much less. Thus, in the last 50 years, both bureaucracies and markets have come to dominate the delivery of healthcare.

The network, a new type of organisation for healthcare

A new type of organisation for the delivery of healthcare is evolving, known as a network:

Networking is a broad concept referring to a form of organized transacting that offers an alternative to either markets or hierarchies. It refers to transactions across an organization's boundaries that are recurrent and involve continuing relationships with a set of partners. The transactions are coordinated and controlled on a mutually agreed basis that is likely to require common protocols and systems, but do not necessarily require direct supervision by the organization's own staff. (1)

Debate often arises about whether the word 'network' is a noun or a verb. The definition of 'networking' in the quotation above summarises the fact that a network is both an entity and an activity, as well as being a gerund, a 'doing' word.

Networks as organisations are different from hierarchies. As emphasised by Wright, networks are not 'top down'.

A network . . . emerges from the bottom up; individuals function as autonomous nodes, negotiating their own relationships, forging ties, coalescing into clusters. There is no 'top' in a network; each node is equal and self-directed. Democracy is a kind of network; so is a flock of birds, or the World Wide Web. (3)

Wright's definition of a network introduces the term 'node', which also helps to differentiate networks from hub-and-spoke organisations. A hub-and-spoke organisation implies that one partner is more important than the others, whereas in a network all the partners – the professor, the generalist, and the patient – are all 'nodes' of equal importance but have different roles.

Networks and teams

Within a bureaucracy, teams play a very important part in delivering care. The importance of good teamwork, particularly multi-disciplinary teamwork, is increasingly being recognised. A new term was developed by Paul Batalden and colleagues at Dartmouth Hitchcock Medical Center – the clinical microsystem – defined as:

. . . the sharp end of care – the places where care is actually delivered in the real world. We call these small frontline systems

of care clinical microsystems. *They are literally the places where patients and families and care teams meet.* (4)

There are, however, important differences between teams, including multidisciplinary teams, and clinical microsystems and networks. Networks differ from teams in at least three ways (see Display 7.1).

Display 7.1

Teams	*Networks*
• Members all work in the same organisation • Communication is primarily face-to-face • One member is usually designated as the person who has bureaucratic authority by the organisation in which the team works	• Members come from different organisations • Face-to-face contact is usually infrequent • It is uncommon for one person to have bureaucratic control

Networks are developed through sapiential authority, that is, an authority based on knowledge, originally defined by Max Weber more than a century ago. Although the leadership of a team can also be strengthened by sapiential or charismatic authority, the designation of one clinician as the clinical director of a department does not necessarily confer all the authority that the person may need. The person designated may not be the most experienced clinician; indeed, they may be the only one willing to do the job. If, however, that person was appointed because they have the right personality for the job, they will be able to generate the necessary charisma.

Types of network

Although networks run primarily on trust rather than hierarchical authority, some of the relationships within a network are governed by formal rules of conduct, or sometimes contracts. The Royal College of Paediatrics and Child Health (RCPCH) defined four types of network depending on the degree of formality (see Box 7.1).

> **Box 7.1 Four types of network identified by the RCPCH (5)**
>
> *Clinical Association:* an informal group that corresponds or meets to consider clinical topics, best practice and other areas of interest
>
> *Clinical Forum:* a more formal group than a clinical association that meets regularly and has an agenda that focuses on clinical topics; there is an agreement to share audit and formulate jointly agreed clinical protocols
>
> *Developmental Network:* a clinical forum that has started to develop a broader focus other than purely clinical topics, with an emphasis on service improvement
>
> *Managed Clinical Network:* includes the function of a clinical forum, but has a formal management structure with defined governance arrangements and specific objectives linked to a published strategy

The evolution of Accountable Care Organisations

In several countries, a more formal split has been established between organisations that pay for healthcare, such as insurance companies, and those who provide healthcare. In NHS England, it is the role of commissioner to pay for healthcare. With the development of this formal split, a type of network is emerging that has a greater degree of bureaucratic, contractual formality than has been the case hitherto. The term for such an organisation in the United States is the Accountable Care Organisation (ACO).

> *ACOs consist of providers who are jointly held accountable for achieving measured quality improvements and reductions in the rate of spending growth. Our definition emphasizes that these cost and quality improvements must achieve overall, per capita improvements in quality and cost, and that ACOs should have at least limited accountability for achieving these improvements while caring for a defined population of patients. (6)*

The term Accountable Care Organisation has been used in the NHS although it has not been generally adopted. There is agreement, however, about the need to develop networks that have more formality than groups of professionals who have a common interest.

One model is for one service to be given a contract to act as the 'prime contractor' or 'prime provider', responsible for involving all the other relevant services and, where necessary, issuing a subcontract. This type of organisation:

- is responsible for ensuring that integrated care is delivered to a defined population within a fixed budget to explicit quality standards and outcomes;
- will need a lead clinician skilled in population medicine, one of whose responsibilities will be to produce an explicit care pathway or care map which most patients should follow through the network.

Another approach is for payers to change the type of contract they use. Traditionally, payers contracted with the main islands in the archipelago of healthcare – hospitals, primary care, community services and mental health services (see Figure 6.1). Such contracts have focused on price and volume supported by a few quality indicators, such as waiting list times. A new approach uses population- and outcomes-based incentivised contracts so that all the relevant clinicians from the different provider organisations are incentivised to work together focused on the needs of, for example, all the people with musculoskeletal disease in a population.

Practical steps in building an effective network for integrated care

When developing a network for integrated care, several variables can influence what it is possible to achieve, including:

- the management style of the health service, for example, has it adopted the principle of the Accountable Care Organisation with a lead contractor;
- the degree to which the network is related to a system of care with a clear, written plan recognised by the principal organisations involved;

- the degree of authority given to the person charged with leading or coordinating the network;
- the support provided to the individual identified as the co-ordinator, for example, has the coordinator been given protected time and secretarial support to arrange meetings, or information scientist support to create a website and a virtual community?

These are the issues that the participating organisations need to discuss. The outcomes of such discussions are likely to be determined by the level of trust the organisations have in one another. There are, however, some general steps that can be taken when building a network to deliver integrated care (see Box 7.2)

Box 7.2 Practical steps in building a network for integrated care, assuming the objectives, criteria and standards have been agreed

- Identify the key constituencies
- Within each constituency, identify the person with power and the person most likely to participate enthusiastically in the network – they may not be the same person
- Involve both patient and carer organisations
- Seek resources for a first meeting of the network; consider asking an influential speaker to the launch
- Ask people to introduce themselves
- Ask participants to work in pairs with someone whom they have not met before to discuss the systems document for five minutes and address the question "What are the priorities that the network should tackle in our first year?"
- Ask people to work in pairs, but this time with a different person whom they have not met before, to address the question 'How could the network be enjoyable and productive?' (For example, how often should we have face-to-face meetings, should we have webinars, is there a place for speakers, either from within the participating organisations or from outside?)

Maintaining the network for integrated care

Networks are dynamic and once set up they need nurturing. The person appointed as network coordinator has the responsibility for maintaining the network. Practical steps to help maintain a network for integrated care are shown in Box 7.3.

Box 7.3 Steps to help maintain the network

- Aim to make all meetings educational, and ensure participants are able to claim points for continuing professional development for either all or part of the meeting
- Buddy up with another network, perhaps not one which is a contiguous competitor, and encourage exchange visits by either the whole network or individuals
- Use the Annual Report as an opportunity for reflection, goal-setting, and motivation
- Encourage the conduct of research projects that involve the network as a whole
- Deal with hostile or unenthusiastic members directly and quickly; enlisting the help of their line manager may be helpful. Always bear in mind the adage: 'When deciding whether to be paranoid or puzzled, choose puzzled – it is much more effective'

Ending the era of primary and secondary care

For the specialist who has responsibility for a population and is developing a network, it is vital to create a culture in which everyone is considered to be of equal importance. This is not always easy to achieve:

- medicine has become split into primary and secondary care, which can be counterproductive when building a system;
- even in the United Kingdom where primary care or general practice is acknowledged as having the same intellectual standing as any secondary care or hospital specialty, a prejudice remains that general practitioners are of lower status.

This prejudice is reinforced when the issue of 'missed diagnosis' in general practice is raised by hospital specialists or of over-use of resources raised by general practitioners.

> *'It was an easy diagnosis. How did those guys miss it?'*
> *Hospital doctor speaking about general practitioners*

> *'Why do they keep doing all these tests? They've lost their clinical judgment.'*
> *General practitioners speaking about hospital doctors*

Although such criticism is sometimes justified, it is usually made by a clinician who is not familiar with the difference between sensitivity and positive predictive value (see Box 7.4). Moreover, this criticism highlights an important consideration in population medicine regarding the different perspectives of clinicians who are providing different types of care for people in the population served:

- the perspective of the clinician in primary care or general practice, who is the first point of contact for the general population;
- the perspective of the clinician in secondary care, who sees only those patients who have been filtered for referral by the clinician who was the first point of contact – these patients represent a subset of the population.

As the prevalence of disease in the general population is different from that in the population subset who have been referred, the positive predictive value for every test is different.

Box 7.4 Definitions of sensitivity and positive predictive value

- *Sensitivity:* the proportion of people with the disease who are identified as having it by a positive test result
- *Positive predictive value:* the probability that a person with a positive test result actually has the disease (7)

Furthermore, the neurosurgeon who says that haemorrhagic stroke is an 'easy' diagnosis because all the patients reaching the service complain of atypical headache in middle age is failing to appreciate that, although almost all of the patients who have had a stroke will report that they had an atypical headache, if every general practitioner referred every patient with atypical headache the specialist service would collapse.

In building a community of practice, it may be more helpful to talk of generalists and specialists, but this terminology could also have pejorative connotations. Although specialists may know more about a particular specialty, it is important to recognise that specialists and generalists are dealing with different subgroups within the whole population served.

When building a system of care and creating a community of practice to work within that system, it is important to encourage a culture change in which people refer to all the clinicians serving a population, and the terms primary and secondary care are made redundant.

Making care pathways

As the delivery of care becomes more complicated, both patients and clinicians can benefit from care pathways, which describe the path a patient with a particular problem usually follows through the network. The term 'care pathways' or 'integrated care pathways' (ICP), however, is used in different ways. A team in Scotland has identified three different meanings associated with the term integrated care pathway (see Box 7.5), and although they believe all three meanings are valid considerations when developing pathways they would argue that only point 3 represents an integrated care pathway and suggest that points 1 and 2 are called 'pathways of care'. (8)

Depicting the care pathway using software such as the Map of Medicine® (see Figure 7.2) helps develop a common understanding of the aims and objectives of the system and contributes to the collective memory of the system. The system of care can be regarded as a neural network, which is based on knowledge.

Box 7.5 Different meanings attributed to the term 'integrated care pathway' (8)

1. The actual care process experienced by each individual patient/client: in the literature, this is represented as a journey in which the patient/client is the traveller

2. Maps that define best practice and the minimum clinical standards or essential components of care for every patient/ client in a given situation: a care pathway is a standard or universal plan for how a patient/client with a particular condition will be treated

3. Physical documentation located at the point of care which may replace traditional records, also called the care pathway: central to the task of patient/client care under the pathway approach, as the care process is clearly presented on the documentation for all those involved to see

---

Resistance to the development of care pathways

There has been professional resistance to the development of care pathways which some clinicians claim will lead to standardisation or 'cookbook' medicine. Although such criticisms need to be addressed, one powerful way to tackle widespread unwarranted variation in clinical practice is through the use of care pathways. In addition, standardisation of certain aspects of clinical care enables the inexperienced clinician to concentrate on an individual patient's anxieties and concerns and to personalise the patient's care, rather than trying to remember which post-operative fluid regime a particular surgeon prefers. Standardisation is particularly important therefore when care is delivered by inexperienced clinicians.

Another reason why standardisation of clinical care has been resisted is because some clinicians see it as a political process.

> *... standardization is a thoroughly political enterprise in at least two ways. First of all, standardization is political in the sense*

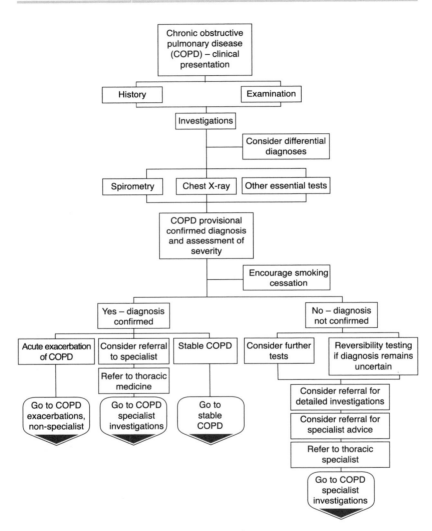

Figure 7.2 The Map of Medicine® page for stable COPD

that the process of standardization is typified by ongoing negotiations between a host of actors, none of whom is in control or oversees all issues that may be at stake. . . . Second, standardization is political since it inevitably reorders practices, and such reorderings have consequences that affect the position of actors (through, for example, the distribution of resources and responsibilities). (9)

Although this view of standardisation can be justified because the implementation of standardisation will affect clinical freedom, to oppose standardisation when there is incontrovertible evidence of unwarranted variation in clinical practice is politically naïve. Clinicians who defend clinical freedom fail to appreciate that there are two types of freedom, distinguished by Isaiah Berlin in his essay *Two Concepts of Liberty* (10):

1. negative liberty, the freedom for every individual clinician to decide on every process of care;
2. positive liberty, the amount of freedom a profession has to decide how much negative liberty its members should have.

Many people who fight for negative liberty fail to see that it is more advantageous to maintain 'positive liberty'. Professional organisations need to be at the forefront of standardising clinical practice, or else, in defence of negative liberty, they will sacrifice positive liberty, that freedom which it is most important to possess.

The way in which pathways are introduced can reduce the level of resistance. For example, when localising a pathway, expressed using the Map of Medicine®, it is important to emphasise that it needs to be adapted for the local population. Some items in the pathway need to be localised, such as the names and contact details of key local services. Some items should not be varied, such as the prescription of a drug which is supported by very strong evidence and national guidance. However, there are often steps in the pathway that can be changed because of some local circumstance, such as the opportunity to offer a patient entry into a randomised controlled trial.

The inevitability of networking

Manuel Castells, one of the intellectual giants of the last 50 years, describes how networks are driving what he calls the Third Industrial Revolution (11). Castells cites the three drivers of this revolution as citizens, knowledge, and the Internet. Following technological developments over the last five years, it is now possible to substitute the smartphone for the Internet. Although Castells' analysis does not include healthcare, it is highly relevant to the development of health services in the 21st century. In this context, the driving forces in organisational development are patients, knowledge and the Internet, all of which interact with one another.

The Internet, by its very nature, promotes networks. It is not merely a passive transmitter of bits of information; it facilitates the creation of knowledge, for example, within healthcare, by allowing instant feedback from patients. The Internet helps to create what has been called a networked information economy.

> *The fundamental elements of the difference between the networked information economy and the mass media are network architecture and the cost of becoming a speaker. The first element is the shift from a hub-and-spoke architecture with unidirectional links to the end points in the mass media, to distributed architecture with multidirectional connections among all nodes in the networked information environment.* (12)

The network as a complex adaptive system

The network will be the dominant type of organisation in the 21st century. In part this is due to the Internet, but it is also due to the recognition that the bureaucracy and the market, dominant types of organisation of the 20th century, have severe limitations. Networks have been referred to as complex adaptive systems: flexible, resilient and evolving, the best example of which is an ant colony (13).

To function as a complex adaptive system, a health service network requires the different types of clinician, who are clear about their respective roles within the network and their responsibilities towards the population served, to work together to increase value for the whole population.

Questions for reflection or for use in teaching or network building

If using these questions in network building or teaching, put one of the questions to the group and ask them to work in pairs to reflect on the question for three minutes; try to get people who do not know one another to work together. When taking feedback, let each pair make only one point. In the interests of equity, start with the pair on the left-hand side of the room for responses to the first question, then go to the pair on the right-hand side of the room for responses to the second question.

- Think of the best clinical network you know and list at least three of the network's characteristics that might explain its success.
- Think of a clinical network you know that does not work well and list at least three of the network's characteristics that might explain its poor performance.
- Imagine you are the Chief Executive of a hospital: what would be your main concerns about the involvement of 'your' clinicians in clinical networks?

References

(1) Child, J. (2005) *Organization. Contemporary Principles and Practice.* Blackwell Publishing. (p. 15).
(2) Perrow, C. (1970) *Organizational Analysis: a sociological view.* Tavistock Publications, London.
(3) Wright, A. (2007) *Glut. Mastering information through the ages.* Joseph Henry Press, Washington DC. (p. 7).
(4) Nelson, E. C., Batalden, P. B. and Godfrey, M. M. (2007) *Quality by Design – A Clinical Microsystems Approach.* John Wiley and Sons.
(5) Royal College of Paediatrics and Child Health (2006) *A guide to understanding pathways and implementing networks.* (p. 9).
(6) McLellan, M., McKethan, A. N., Lewis, J. L., Roski, J., Fisher, E. S. (2010) A National Strategy to put Accountable Care Into Practice. *Health Affairs* 29(5):982.

(7) Gray, J. A. M. (2009) *Evidence-Based Healthcare.* Churchill Livingstone.

(8) NHS Scotland (2008) *A Workbook for People Starting to Develop Integrated Care Pathways*

(9) Timmermans, S. and Berg, M. (2003) *The Gold Standard. The challenge of evidence-based medicine and standardization in health care.* Temple University Press, Philadelphia. (p. 53)

(10) Berlin, I. (1958) *Two Concepts of Liberty, in Four Essays on Liberty.*

(11) Castells, M. (2004) *The Network Society.* Edward Elgar.

(12) Benkler, Y. (2006) *The Wealth of Networks. How social production transforms markets and freedom.* Yale University Press, New Haven and London (p. 212).

(13) Holldobler, B. and Wilson, E. O. (1990) *The Ants.* Springer.

8

ENGAGING PATIENTS

This chapter will:

- describe the benefits and importance of patient engagement;
- analyse different ways in which engagement can improve the quality and increase the value of healthcare;
- describe the importance and dual role of patients' organisations.

By the end of this chapter, you will have developed an understanding of:

- the importance of patient engagement in health service development and delivery;
- how patient engagement can inform the debate about resource allocation and resource constraints;
- how patients' organisations can be supported.

What's in a name: patients or principals?

'Patients, customers, consumers, clients? We just call them punters. Let's face it, they are taking a chance every time they come into healthcare.'

Doctor in Belfast

Patient: there is a move away from using this term; many professionals prefer to use 'citizen'. Alternatively, some professionals prefer to use terms such as 'people with diabetes' rather than 'diabetic patients' to ensure that a person is not characterised by their condition. In this chapter, the term 'patients' will be used as shorthand for people who have, or fear they have, a condition that could be helped by clinical intervention.

Principal: Economists often describe doctors as 'agents' because they act *on behalf of the patient. The doctor (agent) is informed about a patient's health and their treatment options. The patient (principal) is relatively uninformed about these matters and therefore has to rely on the doctor to act in their (the patient's) best interests. A person will employ the services of an agent if they believe that their utility afterwards will be greater than without the help of the agent.* (1)

From a legal perspective also, the patient is the principal, and the professional is the agent.

The new healthcare paradigm

Systems of care offer a new paradigm for healthcare in the 21st century. One of the changes brought in with this new paradigm is a shift from doctor-centred to patient-centred care. If the 20th century was the century of the clinician, the 21st century will be the century of the patient. This shift is one of the most important aspects of the change in paradigm that is currently taking place (see Figure 8.1).

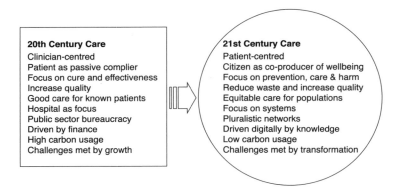

Figure 8.1 The new healthcare paradigm for the 21st century

The implications of this shift are important for all clinicians irrespective of their different roles in relation to the population served, including:

- caring for individual patients;
- managing a service;
- taking responsibility for the whole population of patients.

All clinicians need to adopt a new approach towards patients and understand the benefits that engaging patients will bring. Although one approach is to treat patients as equals in the healthcare transaction, this would not be sufficient because it is now accepted that patients have a major contribution to make to the development and delivery of health services.

The benefits of engaging patients

The main outcome of engaging patients is what is known as 'co-production'.

> *Co-production means delivering public services in an equal and reciprocal relationship between professionals, people using services, their families and their neighbours. Where activities are co-produced in this way, both services and neighbourhoods become far more effective agents of change.* (2)

Co-production can confer benefit in three domains of health service management:

- engagement for performance improvement;
- engagement in decision-making;
- engagement to increase value.

Presenting these domains as a list does not show the potential for interaction and synergy, which is best conveyed diagrammatically (see Figure 8.2).

Rules of engagement

- The clinician responsible for the management of a clinical service has to relate to the patients currently in contact with that service.
- The clinician responsible for population healthcare has to relate to all people in need, irrespective of whether they have been referred or are in contact with the service.

Engaging the patients seen by a clinical service

Throughout the book we have emphasized the difference in managerial accountability for a service, that is to the patients using the service

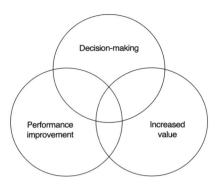

Figure 8.2 The three domains of health service management that benefit from patient engagement

and accountability to a population, some of whose members may be direct users of the service, with others being supported indirectly. This book focuses on the latter responsibility, on population medicine but it is essential to use any opportunities to engage with patients. Engagement with people who are users of a specialist service reaches one part of the population and although it is insufficient by itself as a means of engaging with the whole population in need its potential should be realized by activities such as

- Ensuring a patient or care representative on planning and development groups
- Getting feedback from patients, for example by using www. iwantgreatcare.org or simple suggestion boxes
- Supporting the local branch of the relevant national charity

This is happening in many services and health centres at present but what is not happening is the engagement of people in need who are not yet being cared for by the service. There is a need to engage with the whole population

Engaging with all the patients in the population

It is common to find that the patients being seen by a specialist service are not necessarily those who would benefit most from the service (see Figure 8.3).

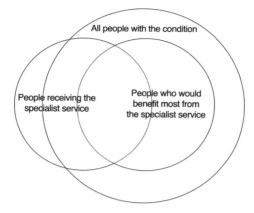

Figure 8.3 The relationship between need and service use

One response to this phenomenon is to increase the size of the specialist service; however, this may not be possible in an era of zero growth. Even if increased resources are available, simply providing more of the same would not maximise value. Instead, action needs to be taken:

To ensure that those people who will benefit most from specialist care are referred, for example, by providing training and guidelines to generalist clinicians for example, domiciliary nurses, community pharmacists and general practitioners.

To increase the knowledge, skill and confidence of all clinicians treating the population so that generalists are able to care for a greater range of patients without referral to specialists; this requires the provision of not only training but also the type of support that can be given easily by telephone and email.

As emphasised in Chapter 2, this approach will increase value from the resources available. It is also an expression of a new culture in which all healthcare professionals, generalists and specialists, work together to care for all the patients with a particular problem. The drawback is that this is a one-way process, from clinician to patient.

To complement the feedback that individual patients are able to give, either about the consultation they have just had or about the service as a whole, is the development of a working relationship between all clinicians and all patients and carers in the population, most easily through the relevant patients' organisations. Many patients' organisations already undertake a dual function (see Figure 8.4):

1. lobbying the body responsible for resource allocation for increased resources for their particular community of patients;
2. helping the relevant service directly, not only by raising funds but also by providing peer-support for newly diagnosed patients and information for patients and carers.

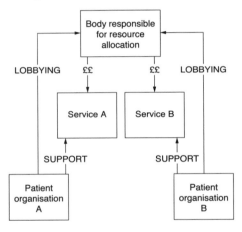

Figure 8.4 The dual role of patients' organisations

Supporting patients' organisations

The clinician practising population medicine can engage with patients other than those in direct contact with the specialist service by supporting the relevant patient organisation (see Box 8.1).

Just as the individual patient is a partner in their care, the community of patients is a partner in the network that delivers services to them.

Box 8.1 Ways in which clinicians practising population medicine can engage with patient organisations

- If a local branch of a patient organisation does not exist, ask the relevant national patient organisation to set one up
- Offer the local patients' organisation practical help, for example, by providing rooms for local meetings
- Offer to attend local meetings to ensure the organisation obtains best current knowledge about evidence from the published literature and about the services provided
- Participate in fundraising events for the organisation

Engaging the public

As resource allocation decisions are concerned with equity, or fairness, rather than efficiency (3), it is important to engage with the population paying for healthcare when making them. There are two main types of resource allocation in which the public may become engaged during decision-making about service provision:

1. The allocation of resources within a service or programme, which is the responsibility of clinicians and managers within each service who must engage with the patients who use that service and their representatives;
2. The allocation of resources across services or programmes, which is the responsibility of those who pay for healthcare or, in NHS England, commissioners, who must engage with the public as well as patients and their representatives.

Although a patient organisation is focused on winning increased resources for the service or programme relevant to their members, it will have implications for other services. Similarly, there may be strong public reaction against proposed change to an individual service, such as the closure of a small but important paediatric service, even when the key healthcare professionals involved are in favour of the change; however, if the service is not closed, there is likely to be a negative impact on other services at the hospital.

If the public are not involved in the whole debate about resource allocation, the focus for argument may fall on one particular 'priority' after another, leading to demands that each should be funded, in the absence of a public appreciation that in allocating resources for one purpose there is an opportunity cost through which resources are denied to another group of patients.

By involving the public, and by definition their political representatives, in the debate and decision-making, payers are able to shift the focus from being held to account for meeting every need to being held to account for the reasonableness of their decision-making (4) (see Chapter 1).

Questions for reflection or for use in teaching or network building

If using these questions in network building or teaching, put one of the questions to the group and ask them to work in pairs to reflect on the question for three minutes; try to get people who do not know one another to work together. When taking feedback, let each pair make only one point. In the interests of equity, start with the pair on the left-hand side of the room for responses to the first question, then go to the pair on the right-hand side of the room for responses to the second question.

- What are the disadvantages of engaging patients and their representatives in the management of services?
- What three points would you emphasise when making a presentation to a group of sceptical clinicians about increased engagement of patients.
- A patient group has nominated somebody to be their representative on a management team. They ask you for guidance about the duties of a 'patient representative' in this situation. Identify five points about the responsibilities this role would involve

---

References

(1) Wonderling, D., Gruen, R. and Black, N. (2005) *Introduction to Health Economics. Understanding Public Health.* Open University Press (p. 100).

(2) Boyle, D. and Harris M. (2009) Discussion Paper: The Challenge of Co-Production. How equal partnerships between professionals and the public are crucial to improving public services. NESTA (p. 11).

(3) Anand, S. (2004) The Concern for Equity in Health. In: Anand, S., Peter, F. and Sen, A. (Eds). *Public Health, Ethics and Equity.* Oxford University Press. p. 15.

(4) Daniels, N. and Sabin, J. E. (2008) *Setting Limits Fairly, Learning to Share Resources for Health.* Oxford University Press. (p. 44)

9

CREATING BUDGETS FOR POPULATIONS

This chapter will:

- discuss how programme budgeting provides a context to encourage decision-making to maximise value;
- describe how to build a budget even if the finance is in different parts of the health service;
- describe how to create a budget even if the financial data are not available.

By the end of the chapter, you will have developed an understanding of:

- all the resources that need to be included in a programme or system budget;
- steps that can be taken to increase value;
- rules of thumb for estimating spend even when no financial data are available.

Budget: The contents of a bag or wallet . . . A statement of the probable revenue and expenditure for the forthcoming year.
Shorter Oxford English Dictionary

The meaning of the term 'a budget' includes other resources in addition to financial resources. A budget is not a synonym for healthcare finance. Thus, the resources available to a clinician practising population medicine are greater than the financial resources of the service for which they may be managerially responsible because the potential resources include the contributions of volunteers, carers and patients (see Figure 9.1).

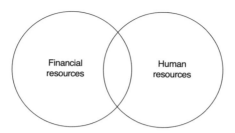

Figure 9.1 The resources of healthcare

It is important for clinicians practising population medicine to be good stewards of all resources irrespective of whether the resources they are responsible for committing are directly charged to their budget (see Figure 9.2). Types of expenditure that tend not to be directly charged to clinical budgets include laboratory tests or imaging.

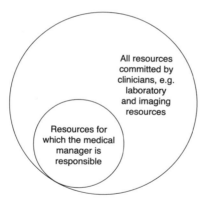

Figure 9.2 Direct and indirect responsibility for resources in a health service

Leadership and budget management

The creation of population healthcare is a leadership and not a managerial task. It is primarily concerned with culture change and not bureaucratic control. The key considerations for clinicians responsible for systems of care are:

1. the population they serve, not just the patients referred;
2. the need to be good stewards of all the resources already available before they bid for increased resources;
3. the need to be part of a community of practice, all of whose members and their resources need to be treated with respect and altruism.

Medical managers usually have responsibility for, and authority over, a delegated budget. As shown in Figures 9.1 and 9.2, clinicians with responsibility for a population need to mobilise both financial and human resources over which they have no direct managerial control. Indeed, such clinicians may not have control over the financial resources for the specialist service in which they work. This is because the role of the clinician with responsibility to and for a population will usually be different from that of departmental manager, particularly if both roles include clinical responsibilities.

The clinician with responsibility for a population has to mobilise the required resources through leadership rather than management: managers are responsible for the day-to-day operation of a service, whereas the leaders are primarily responsible for shaping the culture.

The culture needed to promote population healthcare is shown in Box 9.1. The culture for population healthcare is not the type of command-and-control culture that evolves when a single department or institution pursues a particular target. Although it has been popular for the last few decades, there is increasing evidence that the approach of pressing people to perform well and rewarding them financially if they do so is not only less effective than was originally thought but also has severe adverse effects (1, 2). Furthermore, a culture in which institutions compete with one another for prestige, power and money results in behaviour by which other services are exploited or even deceived.

The model for population healthcare is that of a complex adaptive system, the best example of which is the ant colony. Ants do not compete at the level of the individual: the whole colony works together and different groups of ant within the colony cooperate and make sacrifices for the benefit of the whole. Promoting a culture supportive of population healthcare represents a leadership challenge especially when trying to make the best use of programme or system budgets.

> **Box 9.1 The culture of population healthcare**
> - All the agencies involved are focused on the population to be served, not their own well-being
> - People in one organisation are concerned about possible adverse effects of decisions on other organisations and seek to mitigate them
> - Individuals and individual organisations behave altruistically, that is, they may take decisions or behave in ways that are not advantageous to their particular position in the short term

Programme budgets

A programme consists of a set of systems with a common knowledge base and a common budget. Programme budgeting is a technique that enables personnel in a health service to identify how much money has been invested in major health programmes, with a view to making future investment decisions more rational and have a greater focus on value.

> While the terms 'budgeting' and 'budgets' are normally applied to current and/or future allocations of expenditure, in the context of programme budgeting and programme budgets, it is assumed that they can be applied to past allocations as well. The principle underlying programme budgeting is very simple. If decisions are to be made about broadly defined health-care objectives and priorities – for example, what are the objectives associated with care of the elderly? What relative priorities are attached to the treatment of cancer compared with the prevention of heart disease? – then data should be provided in similarly broad terms to match the nature of the choices. (3)

The NHS in England is fortunate because it has one of the best national programme budget schemes in the world, first initiated in 2002. At the time of writing, there are 23 programme budgets in NHS England, based on the World Health Organization's International Classification of Diseases 10 (ICD10). This information provides the NHS with an opportunity unique among countries with developed economies to identify:

- where resources are currently being invested;
- the value of those investments by relating outcomes to resources;
- the most effective way of investing in health services in future in relation to the needs of the population.

Estimated expenditure for 2010/11 on each programme in NHS England is set out in Table 9.1.

The advantages of programme budgeting are:

- the potential to engage clinicians in discussions about value for money when conventional budgetary procedures have failed;
- increased involvement of clinicians in resource allocation;
- improved information support during decision-making by payers for or commissioners of healthcare;
- the potential to involve the public and patients in decisions about resource allocation.

There are, however, some weaknesses associated with programme budgeting in England (see Box 9.2)

Despite the weaknesses inherent in the programme budgeting scheme for NHS England, the data are very useful. Programme budgeting information enables the clinician responsible for population medicine to improve healthcare for the local population. To ensure the usefulness of the data, however, they need to be:

- reproduced at the level at which resources are actually allocated, for example, in a county like Derbyshire, with a population of 600,000, as well as at national level;
- related to outcome;
- owned by the clinicians who commit the resources;
- further subdivided by systems.

Table 9.1 Programme budgeting estimated England-level gross expenditure for programmes in 2010/11[1]

Programme budgeting category code	Programme budgeting category	Gross expenditure 2010/11 (£billion)
1	Infectious Diseases	1.80
2	Cancers & Tumours	5.81
3	Disorders of the Blood	1.36
4	Endocrine, Nutritional and Metabolic Problems	3.00
5	Mental Health Disorders	11.91
6	Problems of Learning Disability	2.90
7	Neurological	4.30
8	Problems of Vision	2.14
9	Problems of Hearing	0.45
10	Problems of Circulation	7.72
11	Problems of the Respiratory System	4.43
12	Dental Problems	3.31
13	Problems of the Gastro-Intestinal System	4.43
14	Problems of the Skin	2.13
15	Problems of the Musculo-Skeletal System	5.06
16	Problems due to Trauma and Injuries	3.75
17	Problems of the Genito-Urinary System	4.78
18	Maternity and Reproductive Health	3.44
19	Conditions of Neonates	1.05
20	Adverse Effects and Poisoning	0.96
21	Healthy Individuals	2.15
22	Social Care Needs	4.18
23	Other Areas of Spend/Conditions	25.95
Total		107.00

[1] http://www.dh.gov.uk/health/2012/08/programme-budgeting-data/

Box 9.2 Weaknesses in the construction of national programme budgets in NHS England

- Although the cost of drugs prescribed in general practice and the cost of referrals made are assigned to relevant budgets, the cost of primary care professionals' time, principally that of general practitioners, is not assigned to the relevant budgets
- The category 'Other' represents spend not classified by disease programme, and is very large; included within this budget are primary care, education, and the costs of many of the bureaucratic bodies that run the NHS
- Expenditure on education, research and management is not assigned to relevant programme budgets
- Budgets are expressed only in financial terms; the 21.8 million tonnes of carbon produced by the NHS each year should be assigned to programme budgets in a similar way
- Some of the programme budgets have less granularity than others; for example, in the Cancers and Tumours budget, it is possible to identify the amount spent on each of the common cancers, whereas in the budget for Problems of the Respiratory System, although there are sub-budgets for asthma and chronic obstructive pulmonary disease (COPD), the biggest sub-budget is 'Other'; coding will improve as programme budgets grow in importance
- The underlying assumption for programme budgets is that people have a single diagnosis; however, as many people have more than one diagnosis, it is useful to base programme budgets on populations, such as frail elderly people, as well as on conditions (see Figure 9.3)

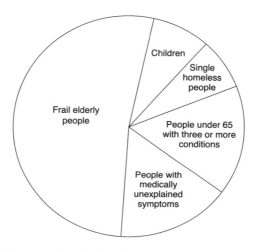

Figure 9.3 Population-based programmes of care

System-specific budgets

Whereas a programme is at the level of Cancers and Tumours, Mental Health Disorders or Problems of the Respiratory System, the system is at a finer level of granularity. To take respiratory health as an example, within that programme there are systems of care for asthma, chronic obstructive pulmonary disease (COPD), and sleep apnoea. Therefore, the person responsible for a population-based programme almost always has an additional responsibility for several population-based systems of care. Furthermore, each of the systems within a programme may be championed by a clinician keen to develop the system for which they are responsible. Thus, the person responsible for a population-based programme not only has to compete with other programmes either to increase resources or to prevent resources being taken away, they also have to deal with competing claims from clinicians responsible for the systems of care within that programme (see Figure 9.4).

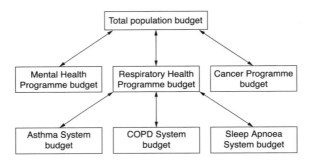

Figure 9.4: Programme and system budgets

People who commission or pay for healthcare must make decisions about the allocation of resources to different programmes, addressing questions such as:

- Should we switch resources from one programme to another?
- Into which programme should we invest new resources?
- From which programme should we cut resources?

Once the budget has been allocated to a programme, however, the clinician practising population medicine has to ask an analogous set of questions.

- Have we got the distribution of resources right among the various systems of care within the programme or should we redistribute?
- If I have to make a cut from one of the services, which should it be?
- If I am able to release some resources, to which of the services should those resources be given?

When practising population medicine, it is essential to be aware of *all* the key resources that are being spent on a particular condition or a group of conditions within the population served, irrespective of which institutions are responsible for the management of those resources. Rarely is a financial budget for a system available at a local level. Usually it has to be created using the framework in Table 9.2. The simplest approach is to prepare an inventory of all the key resources used, and once they have been listed to express the financial costs of those resources; if there are no accurate costings available, then it is important to make an estimate.

Sometimes, it is relatively easy to identify the financial spend and the use of resources on a specific condition if the service is discrete, but in some specialties clinicians will deal with more that one condition during the same clinic, and in primary care the general practitioner will deal with many conditions – from asthma to depression to heart failure to a medically unexplained symptom – during the course of one surgery. It should, however, be possible to estimate to the nearest million pounds what money is spent on a particular condition in a particular population. Estimates for services delivered to subgroups of that population, such as children or frail elderly people, are more difficult but should still be attempted.

The expenditure associated with calculating to the nearest pound the amount of money entailed in the delivery of a service is high. Any service in which an attempt is made to bill every item needs to spend a large amount on administration unless it is a specialist hospital doing only elective surgery on healthy people. The precise costing of a single episode of care, or the precise costing of a whole service, would not justify the level of expenditure on data collection except as a research exercise. Any service that has to deal with emergencies, or admits older people with four or more diagnoses, would face huge costs were it to try to account for every catheter or drip set. One of the joint winners of the Nobel Prize for Economics in 2009, Oliver Williamson, was recognised for his work over the last 20 years, which highlighted the large transaction costs associated with both markets and bureaucracies when they try to achieve greater efficiency through micro-management.

Budget-building: key questions about key resources

The remainder of this chapter is dedicated to outlining the steps that can be taken to build a budget by mapping all the key resources, both human and financial, that are necessary for a system of care (see Table 9.2).

Building a budget, even if precise financial data are not available, is essential; it is better to be accurate than precise. Accuracy allows clinicians to focus their attention and use their clinical knowledge to

Table 9.2 Budget-building: key questions about key resources

Key resource	Comment	Key questions	Key financial issues
Patients	Patients are probably the most neglected resource	• What steps are being taken to provide and support self-care? • Do the patients hold their own records? • Can they request follow-up consultations or telephone advice as they feel they require it, or are they scheduled into regular clinic appointments?	Probably no finance identified for patients; there should be a budget for patient information; if there is none, one should be created
Carers	Carers are another neglected resource	• How heavy is the burden on carers? • Does carer exhaustion play any part in demand on services? • Do carers have all the information they need, including information about access in emergency?	No finance usually identified for carers; as for patients, there should be a budget for carer information
Patient organisations	Patient organisations play an invaluable role in networks of care	• How many national patient organisations are there? • How many, if any, local branches are there of these organisations? • What is the potential for strengthening and expanding their contribution?	Patient and carer organisations can be helped without finance, e.g. by the offer of rooms for meetings, but small grants give a very good return on investment in patient organisations
General practice	There is a high degree of variation in the clinical practice of general practitioners	• What proportion of general practitioners' time is spent on this condition? • What resources do general practitioners feel they lack? • Are there particular general practitioners with special skills or interests who want to do more? • Could general practice trainees be more involved with the service?	The only way to estimate the financial cost of general practice time is to take the percentage of consultations on the condition and use this to calculate the financial cost of general practice input; this estimate is probably not worth the effort required

Community services	Community services may be based in a community services organisation or work as outreach services from a hospital	<ul><li>What is the involvement of: – health visitors; – home nurses; – occupational therapists; – physiotherapists; – podiatrists.</li><li>What constraints do these staff face in delivering high value care?</li><li>Who are the leaders within these professional groups?</li></ul>	Good data on number of visits and work done, but financial cost may have to be estimated by using the percentage of work done on the condition in relation to the total budget of community services
Social care	Social care is a key resource even though it may be supported from another financial stream	<ul><li>How much resource does social care invest in people with this condition?</li><li>What constraints impair social services' ability to be as helpful as the health service thinks they could be?</li><li>In what way could healthcare resources be used to reduce pressure on social care budgets?</li></ul>	Usually very well costed by the local authority
Private care	Private care has more relevance for some health services than others; impacts on health service resources can be both positive and negative	<ul><li>What private sector resources are used by people with this condition?</li><li>Is the impact on publicly funded services negative or positive?</li><li>How could a clearer understanding between sectors improve the value derived from public resources?</li></ul>	The cost per case, or at least the price charged, is usually public knowledge; the number of cases is not
Pharmacists	The knowledge and skills of pharmacists are probably the most under-used in the healthcare workforce	<ul><li>How much hospital or specialist pharmacist time is committed to the programme?</li><li>Is there a pharmacist with a special interest or responsibility?</li><li>Could the specialist pharmacist make an even more valuable contribution?</li><li>How many community pharmacists are involved with patients?</li><li>Could their contribution be more valuable with additional training or specialisation?</li></ul>	It is usually simple to cost whole-time equivalents using pharmacists' salaries

Table 9.2 (*cont.*)

Key resource	Comment	Key questions	Key financial issues
Medication	Medication is often the fastest growing cost	• How many people receive drug treatment? • How much variation is there in prescribing? • Where are generic options available and what proportion of prescriptions are generic? • What proportion of drugs is taken as prescribed?	Usually well documented
Specialist clinics	The term "outpatients" is an outdated 19th century term	• How many clinic sessions are there in the year? • Are all the sessions managed by consultants? • Assuming a 100% attendance rate, how many consultations can take place in these sessions? • Are telephone or email consultations and contacts available?	Much more difficult to find data; clinics may not be charged to each specialist service
Hospital beds	Even though hospital beds are not owned by the relevant specialty, an estimate of bed-days should be included in the inventory	• What is the average duration of stay? • How many admissions take place in the course of the year? • How many bed days are used in the year? • What proportion of hospital admissions were day cases?	Difficult to cost but the finance department are usually able to provide an estimate
Theatre resources	Theatre resources are not applicable to every specialty; they are often difficult to calculate because the relevant operations may be done as part of a long list with other operations	• How many operations were done in the last year? • What was the cost of equipment used in the operations?	The theatre manager can often provide good costings for a theatre session
Imaging	For some diseases, the demand for imaging is growing at a faster rate than that for drugs	• Number of MRIs and rate of increase since previous year • Number of CTs and rate of increase since previous year • Number of other images and increase since previous year • Is there any scope for increasing interventional techniques to reduce the use of other resources?	Some imaging departments have good costings

Laboratory services	More than one estimate may need to be prepared for different types of service, e.g. biochemistry and haematology, depending on the condition	• What are the tests most commonly ordered? • Is it possible to classify the tests as used for either diagnostic or monitoring purposes? • What is the rate of increase in the five most commonly requested tests?	The cost per test may be available but remember to cost the work generated by false-positive test results
Specialist personnel	Specialist personnel are the most valuable and expensive resource	• How many whole-time equivalents of: – nursing staff? – medical staff? – physiotherapists? – occupational therapists? – scientists? – managerial staff? – staff in training?	The cost can be estimated from the salaries of specialist staff
Real estate	Real estate comprises such items as wards, clinics, and offices; at present, real estate is rarely charged to clinical teams, but this will change	• How much space is occupied by the service as sole occupier? • How much space do we share with other services? • Of the space we occupy alone, what proportion of it is not occupied for more than half the time?	Difficult to estimate but can be done by using the proportion of the whole hospital budget that the service represents and then calculating the proportion of the capital value
Information Technology (IT)	Although IT is a consumer of resources, it is also a potential saver of resources	• Does the service have any contracts for IT? • What proportion of the total IT budget is the service responsible for?	The possibility of costing IT depends on the balance of stand-alone IT to the share of general hospital IT
Management and administration	It is essential to maximise productivity in management and administration, but what is the right level of investment?	• Number of whole-time equivalent administrative and management staff • Notional share of central management costs, e.g. human resource departments • Number of whole-time equivalents of professional staff with explicit management duties	Staff wholly employed in the service can be calculated; general overheads can be estimated as 50% of clinical staff salaries

obtain increased value from the resources available by asking the following questions, and answering them honestly.

- Could we reallocate the resources among the services funded by the programme to achieve increased value for the common problems we face?
- Within the budget for each common problem, can we shift resources from lower- to higher-value interventions?
- Of the activities we do, can we reduce the level of one or more to free resources for ?
- Could we reduce the purchase cost of some drugs or equipment?

Thus, value can be increased by addressing these questions and acting upon the answers.

Questions for reflection or for use in teaching or network building

If using these questions in network building or teaching, put one of the questions to the group and ask them to work in pairs to reflect on the question for three minutes; try to get people who do not know one another to work together. When taking feedback, let each pair make only one point. In the interests of equity, start with the pair on the left-hand side of the room for responses to the first question, then go to the pair on the right-hand side of the room for responses to the second question.

- How would you organise your first meeting on population-based planning?
- How should common symptoms such as breathlessness be dealt with in a programme budgeting system that assumes every patient has a diagnosis?
- If you were a commissioner faced by a demand for more resources for cataract surgery, how could you relate this bid to other uses, within an eye service, to which the same amount of resources could be put?

References

(1) Seddon, J. ( ) *Freedom from Command and Control.* [? details]
(2) Gardner, H. K. (2012) Performance Pressure as a Double Edged Sword. *Administrative Science Quarterly,* 57: 1–46.
(3) Mooney, G. H., Russell, E. M., Weir, R. D. (1980) *Choices for Health Care.* The Macmillan Press Ltd. (pp. 10–11).

10

MANAGING KNOWLEDGE

> **This chapter will:**
> - Emphasise the benefits of managing knowledge as carefully as one manages money;
> - Provide a classification of knowledge;
> - Describe what can be done without spending more money to manage knowledge better.
>
> **By the end of this chapter, you will have developed an understanding of:**
> - The difference between tacit and explicit knowledge;
> - The role and responsibilities of the Chief Knowledge Officer;
> - How to realise the potential of librarians;
> - How knowledge from experience can be harnessed.

Toyota is a knowledge business.
President, Toyota Motor Corporation

Toyota plans to introduce two electric vehicles in the United States and six hybrid cars worldwide by the end of 2012.
International Herald Tribune 15.9.2010

Healthcare is a knowledge business

It is clear that healthcare is in the business of improving health, just as Toyota is in the business of producing cars, but few people would realise that Toyota's second dimension was in the business of knowledge. Some people think of healthcare as in the business of real estate – building more hospitals – and some think of it as in the business of technology, such as scanners, drugs and sterilising equipment. However, healthcare is a perfect example of a knowledge business.

Although chief executives of hospitals must manage the real estate, they employ 'knowledge' workers, that is, people who add value because they know more about a particular topic than anyone else in the population. It is knowledge that creates the technology, and knowledge that determines when it should be used for best value.

In most health services, however, knowledge is managed much less carefully than money or buildings. It is relatively easy to discover the name of every estates manager in the NHS, but not the name of every knowledge manager. Indeed, in many NHS organisations, no-one has this responsibility.

Knowledge management responsibilities in population medicine

As knowledge is critically important in achieving good outcomes for patients and in maximising value from clinical services, clinicians with managerial responsibilities (whole- or part-time) should include a responsibility for managing knowledge in their brief, and assume this responsibility if it has not been given to them. Furthermore, as knowledge is shared and exchanged in populations, such clinicians should take responsibility for the management of knowledge for the whole population, not just for those patients in contact with the service.

The management of knowledge for the population is one of the key responsibilities and new skills of population medicine, partly because any service is in competition with other providers. The traditional responsibility towards knowledge management is that all professionals who work within the specialist service should be up to date with best current evidence. This type of responsibility, however, is focussed on self-improvement for a limited number of individuals and could have potentially negative consequences for the care of the population served. In this situation, it is not clear who has overall responsibility for meeting the information needs of the wider community of clinicians serving the population in need (see Display 10.1). Part of the reason for a lack of clarity about who is responsible for managing knowledge for the population is that certain specific responsibilities for information provision may rest with different healthcare professionals.

> **Display 10.1**
>
> **Scenario:** You are a clinician with responsibility for orthopaedic and rheumatology services for a population of 500,000 people
>
> Who is responsible for ensuring that:
>
> - a new general practitioner in the population served knows the referral criteria for back pain?
> - patients are assured that the service provided in their locality serves them better than the service in the neighbouring locality?
> - the hip re-operation rate in your locality is within an acceptable range?
> - older people in the population know about fragility fractures and how they can be prevented?
> - pharmacists and general practitioners know the best-value drug treatment for rheumatoid arthritis?
> - people who make decisions about licensing alcohol understand what they can do to prevent trauma?
> - patients considering knee replacement understand the probability and nature of the risks of the operation as well as they understand the benefits?
> - when surgeons retire, the key lessons they have learnt are captured and passed on?

The roles and responsibilities of three types of clinician in relation to knowledge provision are shown in Table 10.1, however, each role needs to be developed and the coordination among them improved.

Knowledge as a driver for better value healthcare

Manual Castells has described three eras of industrial revolution (2), an analysis that can be applied to the evolution of healthcare.

- The first industrial revolution was driven by empirical commonsense – James Watt did not understand the physics of steam but drew conclusions from the boiling of his mother's kettle; in the first

Table 10.1 Roles and responsibilities for knowledge provision for three groups of healthcare professionals

Healthcare professional and their responsibility to knowledge provision	Action required
General practitioners have a clear responsibility to ensure that: • they have access to best current knowledge; • the patients who attend for consultations receive the knowledge they need.	In a health centre at which there is a team of general practitioners and other clinicians, one clinician should take lead responsibility and adopt the role of Chief Knowledge Officer (see page 00)
Specialist clinicians working in hospitals or mental health services have an important part to play in ensuring that all patients directly supported by the service receive information about their condition, and the probability of the benefit and the harm relating to the different treatment options for their condition	Clinicians who are medical managers of a service should consider the knowledge needs of: • staff in the specialist service; • general practitioners, particularly those new to the locality; • pharmacists in private community pharmacies; • physiotherapists in the community service and private practice; • patients who reach the service.
Directors of public health have a responsibility for delivering public health services to a defined population. Just as it is a public health responsibility to ensure that the population has clean clear water so should it be a responsibility for the public health service to ensure clean clear knowledge? (1)	Directors of public health must ensure that everyone in the local population (including people who do not have a general practitioner) receives the knowledge they need, particularly knowledge relating to how to stay healthy and prevent disease

healthcare revolution, John Snow did not know that the causative agent of cholera was *Vibrio cholerae*, but he did work out that the cases of cholera were linked to water from the Broad Street pump.
• The second industrial revolution was driven by scientific advances; during the second healthcare revolution over the last 50 years, notable scientific advances are hip replacement and transplantation.

- The third industrial revolution is already taking place and is being driven by three forces: knowledge, the Internet and citizens (Figure 10.1); these drivers are also highly relevant to healthcare, and in particular to population medicine.

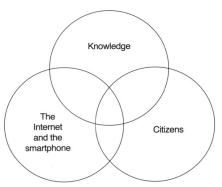

Figure 10.1 Drivers of the Third Healthcare Revolution

It is not common for a clinician to face competition when designing and creating systems and networks for a population but, when trying to ensure that all professionals and patients within a population receive unbiased, clearly presented, up-to-date knowledge, the clinician practising population medicine faces intense competition from the media, particularly the Internet. Key features of the sources of competition to unbiased information about healthcare are shown in Box 10.1.

It is therefore necessary for those who pay for or manage healthcare resources to compete with other sources of knowledge in the knowledge 'marketplace' particularly the Internet.

Classifying knowledge

A simple classification of the different types of knowledge is shown in Figure 10.2. Generalisable knowledge can be classified into several categories (see Figure 10.3).

Box 10.1 Key features of the competition clinicians face when trying to provide unbiased clear up-to-date knowledge about health and healthcare

- Multiple sources of knowledge
- No possibility of controlling what can be found through some sources such as the Internet and newspapers
- No editorial control of content on the Internet
- Newspapers that run campaigns which are not evidence based, e.g. for screening in prostate cancer, especially when celebrities are used as figureheads
- Many patients access the Internet both before and after a consultation
- People who do access the Internet do not always tell their clinician for fear of upsetting the clinician or of being reprimanded

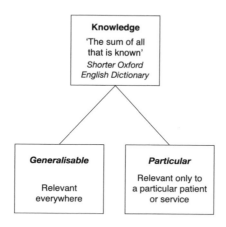

Figure 10.2 A simple classification of knowledge

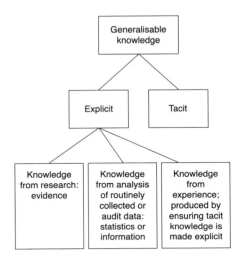

Figure 10.3 Three types of explicit knowledge

Managing different types of knowledge

The management of knowledge involves not only its creation but also its use, both of which require good management. In health services, the management of all types of generalisable knowledge needs to be improved.

Improving the management of knowledge from experience

Tacit knowledge consists partly of technical skills – the kind of informal, hard-to-pin down skills captured in the term 'know-how'. A master craftsman after years of experience develops a wealth of expertise 'at his finger-tips'. But he is often unable to articulate the scientific or technical principles behind what he knows.

At the same time, tacit knowledge has an important cognitive dimension. It consists of mental models, beliefs, and perspectives so ingrained that we take them for granted, and therefore cannot easily articulate them. (3)

Knowledge from the experience of professionals

Of the three types of explicit knowledge, knowledge from experience is the type least well managed. It needs to be created by converting tacit knowledge into explicit forms, for example, by:

- interviewing staff as they leave (exit interviews or knowledge harvesting) to find out what their successor needs to know and how the service could change for the better;
- celebrating successes and profiting from failures by ensuring that there is time for reflection and discussion after a project is finished;
- building a casebook in which people record the outcomes of projects, successful and unsuccessful, and the lessons learned;
- developing partnerships with other services and arranging exchanges so that members of staff can experience different approaches to the same job in different contexts;
- using the Map of Medicine and other software for care pathways to make tacit knowledge explicit in a graphic medium, which is much more accessible for the majority of people.

In addition to these formal techniques of converting tacit to explicit knowledge, learning can be garnered during informal situations. The clinician leading a service needs to create a culture in which discussing the service in a social setting is seen as valuable. The cultural change required is one best described as the transformation to a learning organisation.

> *Peter Senge, who popularized learning organizations in his book* The Fifth Discipline, *described them as places 'where people continually expand their capacity to create the results they truly desire, where new and expansive patterns of thinking are nurtured, where collective aspiration is set free, and where people are continually learning how to learn together'. In a similar spirit Ikujiro Nonaka characterized knowledge-creating companies as places where 'inventing new knowledge is not a specialized activity . . .it is a way of behaving, indeed a way of being, in which everyone is a knowledge worker. A learning organization is an organization skilled at creating, acquiring*

and transferring knowledge, and at modifying its behaviour to reflect new knowledge and insights'. (4)

Within healthcare, the concept of the learning organisation has been promoted by the Institute of Medicine (part of the US National Academies of Science), which produces helpful publications on the topic. The Institute has described the 'Learning Healthcare System' as:

> *The fundamental notion of the learning healthcare system – continuous improvement in effectiveness, efficiency, safety, and quality – is rooted in principles that medicine shares with engineering. The goal of a learning healthcare system is to deliver the best care every time, and to learn and improve with each care experience.* (5)

Knowledge from the experience of patients

The importance of harnessing the knowledge of patients, not only for the purposes of learning but also as part of developing an emotional bond with patients, has been emphasised elsewhere in this book (see Chapter 8).

Improving the management of knowledge from evidence

> *Evidence is generally considered to be information from clinical experience that has met some established test of validity, and the appropriate standard is determined according to the requirements of the intervention and clinical circumstance.* (6)

The definition of evidence quoted above highlights the distinction between evidence from research and evidence from experience: evidence from research requires a 'test of validity'. Both types of knowledge, however, are needed in healthcare. Clinicians worldwide have adopted the paradigm of evidence-based decision-making, and in particular evidence-based medicine. Evidence-based medicine (EBM):

> *... requires the integration of the best research evidence with our clinical expertise and our patient's unique values and circumstances.* (7)

This conception of EBM can be represented graphically (see Figure 10.4).

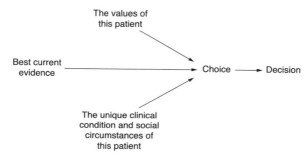

Figure 10.4 The three contributors to informed choice

Evidence-based medicine, however, has been supplemented and complemented by evidence-based management to enable clinicians to incorporate the evidence-based paradigm into clinical practice.

> ... *evidence based management [is the] knowledge of how to put [evidence based medicine] into practice . . . it focuses on the underlying organisational issues that influence how care is delivered. The evidence base comes largely from the social and behavioural sciences, human factors engineering and the fields of health services research. In addition to RCT's [sic] evidence based evidence management uses observational data and methods such as PDCA. (8)*

The medical manager needs to take four steps to facilitate and improve evidence-based clinical decision-making (see Box 10.2).

Improving the management of knowledge from data

Hitherto, the information used by managers has been restricted to finance and activity data. In the 21st century, the priority will be to manage services using information about quality and outcome. Information on quality can be collected through audits undertaken in the institution in which the medical manager works. To obtain information on outcomes, which is essential for the assessment of

---

Box 10.2 Steps to facilitate and improve evidence-based clinical decision-making

1. Support the development of the clinical skills of inexperienced clinicians to enable them to relate the evidence from research to the unique clinical condition and social circumstances of the patient – 'personalised medicine', articulated by Peter Rothwell as a question 'How can I judge whether the probability of benefit from treatment in my current patient is likely to differ substantially from the average probability of benefit reported in the relevant trial or systematic review?' (9). Do not assume that clinicians are better at understanding risk than patients because statistical illiteracy – 'the inability of many physicians, patients, journalists and politicians alike to understand what health statistics mean' (10) is common

2. Provide patients and clinicians with clear up-to-date information

3. Provide patients and clinicians with decision aids to support decision-making when the patient's values are of vital importance, and in particular if consultation time is limited

4. Ensure that best current evidence is delivered when and where it is needed; knowledge delivery should be 'just-in-time', especially as there is an increasing number of staff working part-time. Ways to deliver evidence/knowledge just in time include: (i) embedding it in documents such as laboratory request forms, laboratory reports, or letters to clinical colleagues and patients; (ii) using what are called 'forcing functions' in the safety literature – '. . . *reminders or constraints that suggest or require a certain response from the person using the machine*' (11) – for example, introducing into a process an evidence-based check that a clinician must complete before proceeding

5. Ensure that the evidence base used by each service is regularly updated; an annual update is usually sufficient, except in the case of safety alerts, which should be incorporated and communicated immediately

value, data inputs from the whole system of care are required. For instance, to gain information about the outcome of hip replacement, data are required about:

- the pre-operative health status of the individual;
- the individual's health status three months after the hip has been replaced, long after the patient has left hospital.

Thus, obtaining information about outcomes, including clinical measures and patient-reported outcome measures, requires the co-operation of the entire network of services providing care for the population, and of individual patients seen by the service.

The debate about the relative importance of process and outcome measures has attracted much attention. There is now a consensus that, although both are necessary, in future people who manage healthcare will be held to account not only for the quality and safety of the care they provide to patients but also for the value derived from the resources. There are two ways in which to estimate value:

1. by relating outcome to expenditure;
2. by comparing services, and plotting the position of each service on the value map shown in Figure 10.5.

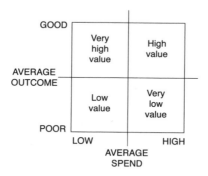

Figure 10.5 The value matrix

It is vital to assess effectiveness in relation to expenditure; indeed, it could be considered negligent not to do so. Even quality improvement, the target of the last decade, needs to be assessed in relation to the cost of achieving any change in the level of performance. Bob

Brook, one of the creators of the quality movement, signalled the end of the quality improvement era in 2010 when he published an article subtitled 'Long Live Increasing Value' (12). The measurement of quality is the means by which institutions can be held to account. The assessment of value, however, requires knowledge to be related to populations and not to institutions.

Improving the management of population-based and not just institution-based knowledge

The principle of population accountability was first developed by Mark Friedman (13). Friedman identified the overlap of, but difference between, outcomes for 'populations' and outcomes for 'customers and communities'. Although Friedman's focus is education, his analysis is relevant to healthcare, especially the relationship between population and performance accountability, which can be directly transferred into a healthcare setting (see Table 10.2)

In an era of resource constraint, it is important to create what has been called 'public value for the population' (14) in addition to providing value for individual patients using the service. The creation of value is critical in a context of increasing demands for transparency from both Government and civil society. The objective of transparency as defined by Manson and O'Neill is to improve levels of trust:

> *Transparency or openness is supplied to improve trustworthiness by exposing misleading claims or failing performance and by creating incentives for institutions and office-holders to be trustworthy, thereby discouraging attempts to play upon others' gullibility in order to gain an unearned reputation for trustworthiness. An expectation of disclosure creates clear incentives for proper behaviour. But by itself transparency does not provide the evidence that is needed to support the intelligent placing and refusal of trust.* (15)

Leadership needs to be provided by the Chief Knowledge Officer.

Table 10.2 The relationship between population and performance accountability

The seven population accountability questions	The seven performance accountability questions
• What are the quality of life conditions we want for our children, adults and families who live in our community? • What would those conditions look like if we could see them? • How can we measure those conditions? • How are we doing on the most important of these measures? • Who are the partners that have a role to play in doing better? • What works to do better, including no-cost and low-cost ideas? • What do we propose to do?	• Who are our customers? • How can we measure if our customers are better off? • How can we measure if we are delivering services well? • How are we doing on the most important of these measures? • Who are the partners that have a role to play in doing better? • What works to do better, including no-cost and los-cost ideas? • What do we propose to do?

The need for a Chief Knowledge Officer

As knowledge is an important resource in any organisation, the management of knowledge requires leadership, and a senior member of staff should be given overall responsibility for managing it. This responsibility can be encapsulated within the role of a Chief Knowledge Officer (16), which was first developed by the private sector in the United States. It is important to emphasise that the Chief Knowledge Officer is a leadership role, not a job. A member of the Senior Management Team, preferably a person directly accountable to the Chief Executive, should be given the responsibility for ensuring that knowledge created and used by an organisation is well managed. If knowledge in the organisation is not well managed, the Chief Knowledge Officer should be given a budget and the authority to mobilise resources to rectify the situation.

In a healthcare setting, the Medical Director is usually the person best qualified to be given the role and responsibility of Chief Knowledge Officer. In turn, the Chief Knowledge Officer can ask each clinical director to take on the corresponding role and responsibility for the relevant directorates. Although it is possible to combine the role and responsibility of a Chief Knowledge Officer with those of a Chief Information Officer, the latter post is usually restricted to the management of data and the production of financial and activity information for management. The typical responsibilities of a Chief Knowledge Officer in a healthcare setting are shown in Box 10.3.

Box 10.3 Responsibilities of a Chief Knowledge Officer in a healthcare setting

- Capturing the tacit knowledge within and about the service and making sure it is used
- Identifying and procuring the sources of evidence that the service requires
- Ensuring that all information for patients is unbiased and clear
- Developing the annual reports for clinical systems and services
- Identifying the wider community of professionals caring for the population served by the service and ensuring their knowledge needs are ascertained and met
- Ensuring the Board and Senior Management Team base their decisions on best current evidence

---

The aim of a Chief Knowledge Officer is to get knowledge into action, an activity increasingly characterised as knowledge translation, defined by the Canadian Institute of Health Research as '*a dynamic and iterative process that includes synthesis, dissemination, exchange and ethically sound application of knowledge*'. (17) In an era when financial resources are constrained, the infinite resource that is knowledge can increase value for the population and for individual patients. (18).

The British Standards Institution (BSI) has produced a *Guide to Good Practice in Knowledge Management* (19), in which are identified the qualities that a Chief Knowledge Officer might need (see Box 10.4).

Box 10.4 Qualities for a Chief Knowledge Officer

- A 'frontline' background
- The ability to command the respect of senior management
- A deep understanding of the organisation's business and culture
- A high level of technological literacy
- A tolerance of ambiguity and the ability to work with minimal structure

---

Directors of public health as Chief Knowledge Officers for health knowledge

On 28 July 2010, through Resolution 64/292, the United Nations General Assembly recognised the human right to water and sanitation, and acknowledged that clean drinking water and sanitation are essential to the realisation of all human rights (20). Knowledge is like water. Everyone has a need for and a right to clean clear knowledge, in the same way that they have a need for and a right to clean clear water.

Ignorance is like cholera, a water-borne disease, it cannot be managed by any one individual; it requires the organised efforts of society. Thus, it is a public health responsibility. The responsibility for ensuring that everyone in the population – professionals, patients and the public – has access to clean clear knowledge could be added to the existing responsibilities of directors of public health. This new responsibility could be discharged through the traditional public health method of needs assessment: by identifying groups whose needs for knowledge are not being adequately met and then through the performance management of Trusts with the main responsibility for delivering knowledge to clinicians and patients who have reached the Trusts' services.

In addition, to ensure that clean clear knowledge is available everywhere, directors of public health could work with:

- the public library service;
- social services;
- the third sector of voluntary and community organisations.

Support for the Chief Knowledge Officer: releasing the librarian's potential

It is not possible for the person assigned the role of Chief Knowledge Officer to fulfil all the tasks required without support. The continuing transformation of the library service, with the advent of digital technology and the capacity to deliver documents to any user electronically, opens up the possibility of releasing some of the librarians' time to become knowledge managers for the organisation, with direct accountability to the Chief Knowledge Officer. The librarian is the most valuable resource in the library, and a librarian's skills are too valuable to be confined to that setting.

Librarians of the 21st century, however, need to supplement their existing skill set and master new skills to enable them to undertake new tasks (see Box 10.5).

Box 10.5 Tasks for 21st century librarians as knowledge managers

1. Teaching critical appraisal to clinicians and managers
2. Knowledge harvesting
3. Managing the storage, updating and distribution of guidelines
4. Identifying the evidence needs of different departments and developing an evidence service for each
5. Coordinating the patient information service

Some of these tasks require the support of colleagues who manage IT.

The type of work required of a knowledge manager in support of the Chief Knowledge Officer is new. It could be funded by increasing the level of investment in library services. Although there is a strong case for such increased investment, even in times of economic constraint, an alternative would be to fund librarian support for the Chief Knowledge Officer by changing the balance of tasks a librarian undertakes, for instance, changing the amount of time spent managing the library, e.g. reducing opening hours by 50%. This strategy would provide an opportunity to support the Chief Knowledge

Officer and create increased value from the knowledge and skills of librarians.

Questions for reflection or for use in teaching or network building

If using these questions in network building or teaching, put one of the questions to the group and ask them to work in pairs to reflect on the question for three minutes; try to get people who do not know one another to work together. When taking feedback, let each pair make only one point. In the interests of equity, start with the pair on the left-hand side of the room for responses to the first question, then go to the pair on the right-hand side of the room for responses to the second question.

- If you were given the responsibility of being Chief Knowledge Officer and the necessary authority, what would be your first three actions?
- How could better use be made of the Internet as a means of managing knowledge for a population?
- If a librarian were seconded to your team or department for one day a week, what would you like them to tackle first?

References

(1) Pang, T. et al. (2006) A 15th Grand Challenge for Global Public Health. *Lancet*, 367: 284–6.
(2) Castells, M. (2009) *The Network Society*. Blackwell.
(3) Nonaka, I. (1991) The Knowledge-Creating Company. USA: Published in *Harvard Business Review* 1991:14–15.
(4) *Harvard Business Review on Knowledge Management* (1987) Harvard Business School Press. (p. 49)
(5) Grossmann, C., Goolsby, A., Olsen L. A. and McGinnis, J. M. (????) The Learning Health Systems Series. Roundtable on Value & Science-Drive Health Care. Engineering A Learning Healthcare System. A Look at the Future. The National Academies Press.
(6) Institute of Medicine of the National Academies (2008) Learning Healthcare System Concepts v. 2008. The Roundtable on Evidence-Based Medicine, Institute of Medicine. Annual Report, p. 5

(7) Straus, S. E., Richardson, W. S., Glasziou, P. and Haynes, R. B. (2000) *Evidence-Based Medicine. How to practice and teach EBM.* (3rd Edition) Elsevier Churchill Livingstone (p. 1).

(8) Shortell, S. M. et al (2007) Improving patient care by linking evidence-based medicine and evidence-based management. *JAMA*, 298: 673–676.

(9) Rothwell, P. M. (2007) *Treating Individuals: from randomised trials to personalised medicine.* Elsevier.

(10) Gigerenzer, G. (2010) Collective Statistical Illiteracy. *Arch. Int. Med.* 170: 468.

(11) Vincent, C. (2006) *Patient Safety.* Churchill Livingstone (p. 202).

(12) Brook, R. H. (2010) The End of the Quality Improvement Movement. *JAMA*, 304: 1831–2.

(13) Friedman, M. (2005) *Trying Hard is not Good Enough: how to produce measurable improvements for both customers and communities.* Trafford.

(14) Moore, M. H. (1995) *Creating Public Value: Strategic Management in Government.* Harvard University Press.

(15) Manson N. C. and O'Neill O. (2002) *Rethinking Informed Consent in Bioethics.* Cambridge University Press (p. 178).

(16) Gray, J. A. M. (1998) Where is the Chief Knowledge Officer? *Brit. Med. J.* 317: 832–3.

(17) Lyons, R. F. (2010) *Using evidence: Advances and debates in bridging health research and action.* Atlantic Health Promotion Research Centre. (p. 12).

(18) Gray, J. A. M. (2008) *Evidence-Based Healthcare and Public Health.* Elsevier.

(19) British Standards Institution (BSI) (????) *Guide to Good Practice in Knowledge Management.*

(20) United Nations General Assembly (2010) Resolution adopted by the General Assembly. 64/292. The human right to water and sanitation. A/RES/64/292. 3 August 2010. Sixty-fourth session. Agenda item 48. http://www.un.org/ga/search/view_doc.asp?symbol=A/RES/64/292 http://www.un.org/waterforlifedecade/human_right_to_water.shtml

11

CREATING AND SUSTAINING THE RIGHT CULTURE

This chapter will:

- define what is meant by culture and subculture;
- explain the relationship of culture to systems and structure;
- discuss the relationship between leadership and culture;
- describe the steps that can be taken to create an appropriate culture for the 21st century.

By the end of this chapter, you will have developed an understanding of:

- how to appraise an organisational culture;
- the part that language plays in shaping and changing culture;
- how to assess the culture of an organisation.

Culture is one of the key components of a health service (Figure 11.1), although the paramount importance of culture in a healthcare setting has been recognised only in the last 10 years. After decades in which those who manage healthcare have been preoccupied with structure and financial regulation and, more recently, quality and safety systems, there is a need to focus explicitly on the culture of a healthcare organisation. In part, this awareness of the importance of culture resulted from the publicity about the banking scandals in 2012. In part, the revolutions in healthcare quality and safety have both led to an appreciation of the role of culture in healthcare organisations.

The quality revolution was adopted from its origins in industry, in particular from Japanese industry. The importance of managing culture, however, increased dramatically after it became obvious that there was nothing particularly 'Japanese' about the 'right' culture

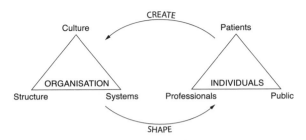

Figure 11.1 The key components of a health service

for continuous quality improvement (although certain aspects of Japanese life make it easier for this type of culture to develop in that country's industrial sector). The safety revolution also started in industry, specifically the aviation industry, although healthcare can be credited for recognising the importance of a safety culture as well as safety systems and of training staff to reduce preventable harm.

The meaning of 'culture'

There are almost as many meanings of the word 'culture' as there are of the term 'leadership'. When multiple meanings of a concept co-exist, it is helpful to take as a reference point a definition that is widely accepted. The definition of culture probably the most highly respected and defensible is by Edgar Schein (1).

The culture of a group can now be defined as a pattern of shared basic assumptions that was learned by a group as it solved its problems of external adaptation and internal integration, that has worked well enough to be considered valid and, therefore, to be taught to new members as the correct way to perceive, think, and feel in relation to those problems. (1)

Another example of a definition for the term 'culture' is used is that by a British team, which highlights that culture influences not only decision-making in an organisation but also the way in which people behave:

. . . assumptions, values and patterns of behaviour within an organization are often termed its 'organizational culture. (2)

It is important to be aware of and recognise the presence of any subcultures within the culture of a health service. The existence of subcultures is determined by three principal influences.

1. The power of national or international cultures relating to a particular specialty: in every country, the culture of a cardiothoracic service is different from that of a paediatric service, and both differ from the culture of a mental health service.
2. The nature of the prevailing leadership, for instance, the culture of a particular cardiothoracic or paediatric service may differ greatly from that of another within the same health service – walking from one ward to another can be like going from France to Italy.
3. The development of countercultures in opposition to the culture created by the official leadership of an organisation. There are two main types of counterculture: formal and informal. The Board of a hospital may regard the trade union as a counterculture, but it has a formal standing. An informal counterculture in a hospital might be one of heavy drinking, or there may a racist subculture.

If multiple meanings of a term do co-exist, it is advisable to take a few minutes at the beginning of any meeting at which culture is discussed to clarify the meaning to be used. Although Edgar Schein's definition can be offered at the outset, it is better to ask participants to work in pairs for two minutes to identify what they believe to be the key points in the definition of culture. For the majority of such discussions, a sufficient number of 'hooks' will be identified for the Schein definition to be adopted by the group.

When initiating the discussion, by way of introduction, it can be helpful:

- to use the commonsense and commonplace definition of culture as 'the way things are done around here';
- to encourage people to reflect on different wards, hospitals or health centres in order to identify elements of culture that may be obvious when we walk into those environments.

Assessing culture

In *Language, Truth and Logic*, A. J. Ayer emphasised that although words could be used to explain meaning, another approach was through measurement (3). Ayer said that:

> . . . *the meaning of a proposition is determined by the observations one would make to confirm or refute the truth of that proposition.*

Propositions such as 'We value diversity' or 'We have a culture of patient-centred care' are commonplace, but how can their truth be determined? There are three main approaches to appraising an organisation's culture.

1. Reading the documents produced and other platforms, e.g. the prospectus or brochure, leaflets for patients, the annual report and the website: such documents reflect the expressed culture, explicitly, through what is articulated, and implicitly for what is absent or lacks emphasis – documents and other platforms, however, are not the only source of information about a culture, and they are probably the least reliable even though a great deal of thought has gone into their production;

2. Observing what Edgar Schein called 'the artefacts of an organisation' (see Box 11.1), which tend to be related to the physical environment: this approach is more likely to produce reliable results than document analysis because less thought has gone into managing the impression organisational artefacts will make on an outsider; however, the physical environment of a service is a fairly coarse measure of culture, and it may be more fruitful to observe and assess staff behaviour not only towards patients but also towards one another;

3. Listening to people who work in or use an organisation: listening is a way of collecting knowledge derived from experience, which can be a rich source of information for culture change. Anthropologists seek out people they call 'informants', namely, knowledgeable insiders who are willing to be interviewed; however, an informant's account may be biased, and the reasons for bias may not be

revealed to the enquirer. Furthermore, the process of listening and observing can change how people behave or what they say, depending on the status of the enquirer and the informant's perception of the purpose of the enquiry.

Box 11.1 Examples of artefacts in a health service organisation
- Are the patient toilets as clean as the staff toilets?
- Is the waiting room decorated in the same way as the Board Room?
- Does the Chief Executive have a designated car-park space close to the front door of the hospital?

Although it is becoming common for Chief Executives in the business sector to visit frontline operations unrecognised, this method of observing organisational culture is more difficult in the health service because in a hospital a Chief Executive is more likely to be recognised by frontline staff.

Mutual learning

It is difficult to learn about the culture in which one works because any culture institutionalises those who work within it. One way to circumvent this difficulty is to take a mutual learning approach. Apply the 'buddy' system and work with someone in another organisation so that each person can act as the key informant about the culture of the other's organisation. A simple template that can be used for reporting these findings (see Display 11.1); it can also be used within your own organisation. Without reflecting on culture change, improvement is not possible.

Culture and leadership

Culture and leadership are inter-related:

> *When we examine culture and leadership closely, we see that they are two sides of the same coin; neither can really be understood by itself. If one wishes to distinguish leadership*

Display 11.1

Method of appraisal	*Observations*
Reading • What struck me about the culture of this organisation from reading its documents? • What impressed me favourably? • What was missing? • What dismayed me?	
Looking • From my observations, were there any signals about the way in which this organisation regards its staff and its patients?	
Listening • When speaking with people: • What did I learn about the culture of the organisation? • Did what I hear differ from what I read in the documents?	

from management or administration, one can argue that leadership creates and changes cultures, while management and administration act within a culture. (4)

This principle is very important to successful organisations like Toyota because:

An organization's culture defines what goes on in its workplace. Loosely defined, culture is the soft, imprecise, fuzzy stuff of everyday life. Within any company, it is what people think and believe and what drives daily priorities. Leadership and a company's culture are inextricably intertwined. (5)

Despite the multiple meanings of the words 'culture' and 'leadership', there is a common thread among them: many of the definitions emphasise that leaders shape culture whereas managers work within it. For the clinician with an interest in population medicine, being a leader and therefore shaping culture is part of the job.

Creating a new culture

Clinicians in leadership positions have a responsibility for changing all aspects of culture.

The shift in healthcare provision from a paradigm in which the concern is with those patients in contact with a service to one in which the concern is for the population served requires a considerable cultural change. A culture with the whole population as its concern exhibits the characteristics shown in Box 11.2.

Box 11.2 Characteristics of a healthcare culture concerned with the population served

- In documents describing the service, there are frequent references to the population served, and not only reports about the quality of care delivered to the proportion of the population in contact with the service but also about the whole population in need, the level of unmet need, and degree of variation in referral rates to the hospital service according to referring practice and socio-economic group of patient.
- Maps are the artefacts that indicate whether a service is concerned with the population. Although maps are rarely visible in hospitals, the service providing care for a population will have numerous maps on display, which provide a key source of information for a population-based health service: for example, maps showing isochrones of the time taken to travel to the hospital from different housing estates in the locality, subpopulations in which there is a high incidence of disease or from which there is a high referral rate. The identification of variation often reveals cultural differences.

This shift in paradigm, however, is one change among several that need to take place if the culture of healthcare organisations is to be transformed from that which was appropriate for the 20th century to that which is appropriate for the 21st century. The various shifts in health service culture that need to take place are summarised in Figure 11.2.

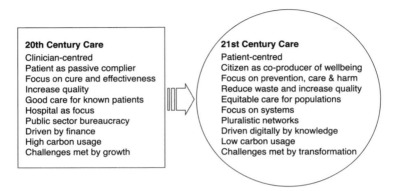

Figure 11.2 The transformation in 20th century healthcare culture to meet the needs of the 21st century

Creating a culture of respect

It is common for clinicians in specialist services to speak with disrespect of clinicians in generalist service, often without experience of having worked in general practice:

> *'I can't think why we don't see more stroke patients. It is a dead easy diagnosis to make – atypical headache in someone of middle age.'*

This specialist, however, has failed to understand an important epidemiological distinction between the sensitivity of a test and its positive predictive value. To the specialist neurosurgeon, the diagnosis is easy because 90% of people who have a stroke of a certain type report this history; however, if general practitioners referred every middle-aged person with atypical headache, the specialist service would be flooded because the positive predictive value of that collection of symptoms is much lower in general practice.

There is a need to move towards a culture in which clinicians in specialist services speak with respect of clinicians in the generalist service because in population medicine all clinicians are of equal standing although they may perform different jobs.

The influence of leadership

Any leader influences culture through what they say and, importantly, through the way in which they behave. For clinicians leading a service concerned with the population served, it is essential to control:

- the editorial content of any documents produced;
- the appearance of buildings relevant to the health service and the environment in which care is provided.

When embarking upon culture change, these aspects of the service convey messages about the organisation's culture, not only to the population served but also to the wider general public.

It is important to be explicit about culture. Ten years ago it would have been rare to discuss the culture of an organisation, whereas now it is common and should be universal. Although the leaders of an organisation must be aware of their behaviour, but they also need to think more about the language they use because language is the dominant determinant in the culture of an organisation. It is also the main way in which culture is conveyed to people who come into contact with the organisation or people who join it. Although the concept of an organisation's 'culture' can sometimes seem nebulous, there are discrete explicit steps that can be taken to influence culture by shaping the language used and the concepts that prevail.

Although the behaviour of the leadership is important in creating a new culture, or in shaping an existing culture, it is necessary to complement behaviour at a leadership level with measures to ensure that people are cognisant of the culture change and act accordingly.

The role of language

When creating a new culture, it is important to examine the language used in an organisation. It is particularly helpful to identify:

- terms that should not be used, such as 'bed blocker';
- terms that need to be used consistently because they are important

to the development of a common set of principles and assumptions, e.g. 'quality' and 'efficiency'. If a term is in common use, it is likely that it has multiple meanings, even within a small management team.

Questions that can be used to identify whether there is a need to create a common language and a set of shared concepts for an organisation are shown in Box 11.3.

Box 11.3 Questions to ascertain whether a common language is needed in an organisation

- If all the key people in the organisation were asked to write down what they meant by patient-centred care, how consistent would the answers be?
- If the leadership team were asked to write down what they meant by the term 'value' and how the meaning differed from that of 'quality', what would they write?
- If all the lead clinicians were asked to describe what they understood by the terms 'inappropriate' care and 'optimal use of resources', how diverse would the answers be?

Language is also shaped by the concepts expressed in books and articles. In addition to a conventional journal club, it would be helpful to establish a 21st Century Book Club. In this type of book club, it is not necessary for everyone to have read the book; instead, the person who has read a book which they regard as important, or has been important to them, describes the key messages as a basis for discussion and reflection.

'Culture eats strategy for breakfast' is the traditional management proverb. More than that it eats structural reorganisation for lunch, dinner and afternoon tea!

> **Questions for reflection or for use in teaching or network building**
>
> If using these questions in network building or teaching, put one of the questions to the group and ask them to work in pairs to reflect on the question for three minutes; try to get people who do not know one another to work together. When taking feedback, let each pair make only one point. In the interests of equity, start with the pair on the left-hand side of the room for responses to the first question, then go to the pair on the right-hand side of the room for responses to the second question.
>
> - How well does your website reflect your official culture?
> - If a colleague from another service or hospital were to visit your facility, which aspects of culture would be viewed favourably and which would be viewed unfavourably for an organisation that claims 'to put patients first'?
> - What book or individual has had the greatest influence on your work in healthcare, and why?

References

(1) Schein, E. H. (2004) *Organizational Culture and Leadership.* John Wiley & Sons Inc. (p. 17).

(2) Mannion, R., Davies, H. T. O., Marshall, M. N. (2005) *Cultures for Performance in Health Care.* Open University Press. (p. 1).

(3) Ayer, A. J. (1935) *Language, Truth and Logic.* Penguin.

(4) Schein, E. H. (2004) *Organizational Culture and Leadership.* John Wiley & Sons Inc. (pp. 10–11).

(5) Morgan, J. M. and Liker, J. K. (2006) *The Toyota Product Development System. Integrating people, process, and technology.* Productivity Press, New York, pp. 217, 218.

CODA

THE NEW PARADIGM: POPULATION AND PERSONALISED HEALTHCARE

For the last four decades the paradigm of healthcare has focused on effectiveness, quality, and safety, primarily involving clinicians and institutions. But a new paradigm is emerging driven by the economic crisis, the Internet and, to a lesser degree, the human genome project. The primary focus is now on value for populations and individuals.

It is surely a major failing that we cannot answer simple questions such as:

Is the service for people with seizures and epilepsy in Alberta better than in Queensland?

Is the prevention and care of liver disease services better in Wales or New Zealand?

Is care for people with bipolar disorder better in Lombardia or Andalucia?

Even within one country which claims to have a National Health Service, questions relating to most common diseases cannot be answered, such as:

Is the service for people with seizures and epilepsy better in Manchester than in Liverpool?

How many liver disease services are there in England, and how many should there be?

Which service for frail elderly people in the London area provides the best value?

Which service for people with bipolar disorder improved most in the last year?

We know to the nearest pound what we spend on every hospital in the world but not even to the nearest one hundred million pounds what we spend on epilepsy or breathlessness. We need personalised healthcare to maximise value for individuals and population healthcare.

Population healthcare focuses primarily on populations, defined by a common need, which may be a symptom such as breathlessness, a condition such as arthritis, or a common characteristic such as frailty in old age. It does not focus on institutions, specialties, or technologies. Its aim is to maximise value for those populations and the individuals within them, and clinicians practising population medicine can and must play a leading part in its creation.

Index

INDEX

laboratory services, 153
language, 90, 183–4
law
 of diminishing returns, 18, 30
 of undiminished harm, 31
lead consultant/clinician responsibilities, 120
 common language and, 184
 job description, 16
leadership, 20–1, 89–90, 141–2, 179–81, 183
 budget management and, 141–2
 culture and, 20–1, 142, 177, 179–81, 183
 development, 19
 knowledge requiring, 168, 169
 need, 20–1
learning, mutual, 179
learning organisations, 163–4
liberty, clinical, 127
librarians as knowledge managers, 172–3
listening in culture appraisal, 178–9, 180
liver disease, 102, 103
 see also hepatology
lobbying (by patient organisations), 136
local sourcing, 75
London School of Economics tool for
 resource allocation, 42
looking/observation in culture appraisal, 178,
 179, 180
lower-value care/activities/interventions, 18,
 28–33, 40, 43, 44, 46, 47, 58, 61
LSE tool for resource allocation, 42
lung (pulmonary) disease
 chronic heart and, 'flu vaccination, 88
 chronic obstructive (COPD), 15, 41–2, 126,
 146, 147
 see also respiratory (disease) services

Managed Clinical Network, 119
management and administration, 96–7, 120
 development, 19
 of knowledge see knowledge
 as resource, 153
 of resources see resources
 staff reduction, 60–2
 time waste, 61–2
 see also medical management
map(s), 125, 181
Map of Medicine®, 15, 124, 127, 163
 COPD, 126
marginal analysis, 36, 38, 52
 within-system, 41
markets, 116, 117, 149
matrix management, 96–7

medical accidents and errors see accidents;
 errors
medical director as Chief Knowledge Officer,
 169–70
medical leadership see leadership
medical management and managers, 4, 5, 6, 7,
 142, 159, 165
medical problems, complex (in treatment)
 distinction from complicated problems, 14
 work undertaken by patients with, 64
 see also ill-health
medications see drugs
meetings about systems of care
 selection of criteria to monitor objectives,
 109
 standard-setting, 111
mental health services, 13, 90, 94, 120, 177
moral meaning of value, 25
motion, waste of, 58
motivation of staff with sustainability, 73–4
motor neurone disease, 101
muda (Japanese for 'waste'), 57
musculoskeletal services (incl. orthopaedics
 and rheumatology)
 programme/system, 99
 responsibilities, 158
mutual learning, 179

National Health Service (NHS)
 patient–doctor contractual arrangement, 3
 programme budgets, 143–4
 weaknesses in construction, 146
 sustainability and, 70–3
National Institute for Health and Clinical
 Excellence (NICE), 45
national screening programmes see screening
 programmes
'necessary' procedures, 28, 30
needs
 individual patient, relating evidence to, 39,
 48
 supply/service use and, relationship
 between, 9, 135
negative liberty, 127
negotiating with payers and commissioners,
 34–8
networks (to deliver systems), 114–29
 as complex adaptive system, 128–9
 defining, 117
 inevitability, 128
 maintaining, 122
 practical steps in building, 120–1